PLASMID

Edited by **Munazza Gull**

Plasmid

http://dx.doi.org/10.5772/intechopen.71424
Edited by Munazza Gull

Contributors

Noboru Sasagawa, Angel Oñate, Munazza Gull, Sondos El-Baz, Ahmed AlHejin, Huda Al Doghaither

Notice

Statements and opinions expressed in the chapters are these of the individual contributors and not necessarily those of the editors or publisher. No responsibility is accepted for the accuracy of information contained in the published chapters. The publisher assumes no responsibility for any damage or injury to persons or property arising out of the use of any materials, instructions, methods or ideas contained in the book.

First published in London, United Kingdom, 2019 by IntechOpen
IntechOpen is the global imprint of INTECHOPEN LIMITED, registered in England and Wales, registration number: 11086078, The Shard, 25th floor, 32 London Bridge Street
London, SE19SG – United Kingdom
Printed in Croatia

British Library Cataloguing-in-Publication Data
A catalogue record for this book is available from the British Library

Additional hard and PDF copies can be obtained from orders@intechopen.com

Plasmid, Edited by Munazza Gull
p. cm.
Print ISBN 978-1-83880-237-0
Online ISBN 978-1-83880-238-7
eBook (PDF) ISBN 978-1-83881-126-6

We are IntechOpen,
the world's leading publisher of
Open Access books
Built by scientists, for scientists

4,200+
Open access books available

116,000+
International authors and editors

125M+
Downloads

Our authors are among the

151
Countries delivered to

Top 1%
most cited scientists

12.2%
Contributors from top 500 universities

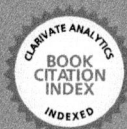

Interested in publishing with us?
Contact book.department@intechopen.com

Numbers displayed above are based on latest data collected.
For more information visit www.intechopen.com

Meet the editor

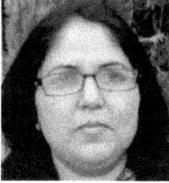

Dr. Munazza Gull is currently working as an associate professor in the Biochemistry Department, Faculty of Science, King Abdul Aziz University, Jeddah, Kingdom of Saudi Arabia. She graduated (MSc Plant Sciences) from the University of Agriculture, Faisalabad, Pakistan, in 1999. She received her MPhil degree in Microbial Plant Sciences from the same university in 2002 and her PhD in Biotechnology in 2008 from the National Institute of Biotechnology and Genetic Engineering Faisalabad, Pakistan/Quaid i-Azam University, Islamabad, Pakistan; she also worked as a researcher for many years in the same institute. She has experience in Microbial Biotechnology and plant-microbe interactions and previously worked with rhizobacteria, biocontrol, integrated disease management, and secondary metabolites/bioproducts/antimicrobial compounds production. Her research interests are now focused on DNA/protein finger printing in human disease management, molecular genetics, environmental/soil/water microorganisms, and phytological/industrial/biomedical productivity potential exploring in both microorganisms and plants.

Contents

Preface

Plasmids are circular or linear extrachromosomal replicons, which are found in many microorganisms in the domains *Bacteria*, *Archaea*, and *Eukaryota*. Also, plasmids are important vehicles for bacterial communication of genetic information, facilitating rapid evolution and adaptation abilities seen in bacteria. In addition, plasmids function as important tools in manipulating and analyzing microorganisms through the introduction, modification, or removal of target genes. In general, plasmid genomes include a backbone of core genetic loci, which are conserved among related plasmids of the same family and associated with key plasmid-specific functions, for instance, replication and mobility. It is by appreciating the genetic independence of these elements that we can understand how they have played a central role in bacterial evolution and in the emergence of molecular biology as the most exciting area of science.

The book opens with the Introductory chapter focusing on the early introduction, double genetic system, lifestyle, and typing of plasmids, reviewing important events and discoveries that have propelled the field forward. The first section of the book details specific plasmid diversity systems, drug resistance, and purification of analytical techniques. The second section includes plasmid optimization and expression and the use of genomic approaches for the study of recombinant proteins. In the last chapter, the use of plasmids as genetic tools and their applications in ecology and evolution are addressed.

This book has been designed for students, researchers, and academicians who are interested in plasmids and their multivariate uses in numerous fields of science.

Most of all, I owe my gratitude to all my expert coauthors, who contributed to this book and helped me gather recent plasmid information in a single volume.

Dr. Munazza Gull
Associate Professor
Biochemistry Department
Faculty of Science
King Abdul-Aziz University
Jeddah, Saudi Arabia

Plasmids Insights

Chapter 1

Introductory Chapter: Preface to Plasmids

Munazza Gull and Sondos El-Baz

Additional information is available at the end of the chapter

http://dx.doi.org/10.5772/intechopen.78673

1. Bacterial double genetic system leads to genetic diversity and evolution

Bacterial genome has unique dynamics, which evolve through a series of evolution. As the result of this evolutionary selection, bacteria have two genetic systems that are chromosomal and extrachromosomal genome. This genetic diversity is the cause for wide range of bacterial adaptation under diverse conditions. Bacteria get this genetic diversity through three processes that are mutation, recombination, and horizontal gene transfer (HGT). Both mutation and recombination is the natural alternation of genes, which has very little part in evolution but horizontal gene transfer alters the genes across the species, and this horizontal gene transfer totally depends on availability of extrachromosomal genome and good environmental conditions. The common mean of horizontal bacterial gene transfer happened through extrachromosomal DNA that is commonly called plasmids [1]. Plasmids are defined as circular or linear extrachromosomal replicons, which serve as important tools in manipulating and analyzing microorganisms through introduction, modification, or removal of target genes found in most bacteria. Plasmids are involved in pathogenicity, host specificity, resistance to antibiotics, and ultraviolet (UV) radiation. In addition to that, they function as toxins and hormones. Popular uses of plasmids are biotechnology and pharmaceuticals. In this chapter, we discussed plasmids as general classification, lifestyle, and role of plasmids playing in different areas of scientific importance. Plasmids modes of transfer, types, properties, and its usefulness for living organisms are also included briefly.

1.1. Plasmids

Plasmids are circular or linear extrachromosomal replicons, which are found in many microorganisms in the domains *Bacteria*, *Archaea*, and *Eukaryota*. Also, plasmids are important vehicles for bacterial communication of genetic information, facilitating rapid evolution and adaptation abilities seen in bacteria [2]. In addition to that, plasmids function as important tools in manipulating and analyzing microorganisms through the introduction, modification, or removal of target genes [3, 4]. Plasmids are harbored by prokaryotic cells where they replicate independently from the chromosome. In addition to that, plasmids are considered a major driving force in prokaryotic evolution since plasmids can be transferred between cells, making them potent agents for meditating lateral gene transfer. Not only they speed up host evolution through the supply of new functions as in antibiotic resistance, but also via variation in copy number that may lead to increased gene expression level and mutation supply rate [5]. In general, plasmid genomes include a backbone of core genetic loci, which are conserved amongst related plasmids of the same family and associated with key plasmid specific functions, for instance: replication and mobility. Plasmids act as efficient vectors of horizontal gene transfer (HGT) [6]. Plasmids were discovered at first in enteric bacteria from late 1950s and recorded as an increased relation in antibiotic resistance [7].

2. Classification

Classification of plasmids is essential for identifying newly isolated plasmids. Plasmids information is important in effectively using them as genetic tools for microbial engineering, detecting, isolating, and identifying new types of plasmids in environmental samples. Known plasmids are having available, complete sequence were classified by their host and replicative or transfer systems [8]. Classification is done according to a typing scheme providing useful insights into the epidemiology of plasmid-mediated antibiotic resistance, for instance: studying the plasmids types' composition can determine whether an antibiotic resistance epidemic is driven by diverse plasmids or one plasmid type [9]. Since plasmids are key in spreading antibiotic resistance, many classification schemes have been developed for epidemiological tracking [10–12].

3. Plasmid lifestyle

Plasmid lifestyle is determined by several traits from them are mobility, stability, and indispensability, which differ in magnitude. Transitions between lifestyle, invasion, host range, and plasmid resistance as well as adaptation are caused by the interplay between plasmid traits and host biology. Mobility and indispensability are essential in plasmid ecology; however, plasmid stability is more relevant for long-term plasmid evolution.

4. Role of plasmids

4.1. Pathogenicity and host specificity

Genes involved in pathogenicity and host specificity are categorized in two main groups: a virulence, virulence, and genes involved with a type III protein secretion system. Virulence genes, with notable exceptions are chromosomally encoded. Type III secretion systems, present in many animal pathogens, determine the production of a pilus-like structure, which delivers certain protein products inside plant cells. Those avr genes that have been described are evenly divided between plasmids and chromosomal locations. Avirulence genes have the ability to induce an hypersensitivity reactions (HR) in plant hosts, which carry a matching gene for resistance (R), the so-called gene for gene theory.

4.2. Toxins

Phytopathogenic bacteria produce a variety of toxins, which affect the host plant causing chlorosis and stunting. Genetic determinants for coronatine, one of the toxins are generally located on plasmids. Coronatine is a polyketide, coronafacic acid, coupled by an amide bond to a cyclopropyl amino acid, and coronamic acid.

4.3. Hormones

A number of phytopathogenic bacteria cause outgrowth in their plant hosts, known as knots or galls, for instance, first strain *P. savastanoi* pv. savastanoi affects olive (*Olea europea*), leading to losses for olive in particular. The strains are host specific so the Indoleacetic acid (IAA) genes occur on plasmids in oleander strains, they are chromosomally located in ash and most olive strains (IAA, synthesized in bacteria via indole acetamide and genes involved are found on the T-DNA of Agrobacterium tumefaciens is a plant growth regulator that affects cell proliferation).

4.4. Copper and antibiotics

Plasmid-borne resistance to copper has been found in several pathogenic bacteria, including *Xanthomonas campestris* pv. vesicatoria pathogenic on pepper (*Capsicum annuum*), in *Pseudomonas syringae* pv. syringae pathogenic to fruit trees, and *Pseudomonas syringae* pv. pathogenic to tomatoes and crucifers.

Resistance to streptomycin (Sm) was detected in the pathogen *Pseudomonas syringae* pv. papulans and a number of Gram-negative bacteria present in apple orchards in USA. Copper resistance is often linked to streptomycin resistance, and dual resistance to these bactericides was detected on conjugative plasmids, which range in size from 68 to 220 kb.

4.5. Resistance to UV radiation

Not only *P. syringae* pathogens exist as epiphytes on plant leaves, but also it is essential in spreading pathogens and developing diseases under certain environmental conditions. One aspect of life on surfaces exposed to sunlight is the effect of UV-light, which is in two groups UV-A (320–400 nm) and UV-B (290–320 nm). Since UV-A has longer wavelength, such exposure causes indirect damage to DNA via generation of chemical intermediates such as reactive oxygen species. On the other hand, UV-B causes direct damage to DNA by forming DNA photoproducts [7].

5. Plasmid typing schemes

Plasmid typing is essential for the analysis of evolution, epidemiology, and spread of antibacterial resistance [13]. Plasmids are typed according to Southern blot hybridization using replicons from plasmids of various incompatibility groups such as probes. On the other hand, this method is limited by probe cross-hybridization amongst closely related replicon sequences [14]. Polymerase chain reaction (PCR)-based replicon typing (PBRT), where plasmids are typed according to various replicon sequences, is less laborious and shows higher specificity in detecting replicons [15].

Concerning Gram-negative bacteria, PBRT schemes, which target replicons found in *Enterobacteriacae* and *Acinetobacter baumannii* plasmids are available [16]. However, a PBRT scheme for plasmids of Gram-positive bacteria has been developed focusing on enterococcal [17] and staphylococcal [18] plasmids.

6. Mode of plasmid transfer

Plasmids enter either by active or passive mechanisms. As known, genetic information encoded in a self-replicating extrachromosomal DNA (plasmid) of bacteria is transferred across three processes: conjugation, transformation, and transduction [1].

6.1. Conjugation

This first stage requires cell to cell contact of donor and recipient cells along with DNA metabolism of donor cell. The first step, DNA covalently linked to recipient, is initially transported in a passive manner, trailing on the relaxase, where pilus helps in transporting DNA across several membrane barriers in recipient cell. The second step is active pumping of the DNA to the recipient using the already available T4SS transport conduit. Such stage is known as the active invasion mechanism since the proteins in the conjugative transfer are encoded by plasmids [5, 8].

6.2. Transduction

The second process represents plasmid-mediated gene transfer in bacterial community through bacteriophages, which are viruses affecting bacteria. Transduction is of two types: generalized or specialized. Generalized transduction is the ability of transducing any gene into bacterial chromosome. On the other hand, specialized transduction is done particular genes. Plasmid invasion by membrane vesicles (MVs) has been documented for both Gram-positive and Gram-negative bacteria. In addition to that, MVs mediate interspecific plasmid invasion as in *Acinetobacter baylyi* and *Escherichia coli* [19]. Plasmid transfer through nanotubes between cells was reported only for *Bacillus subtilis* [5, 8, 20].

6.3. Transformation

It is the most common method for transferring bacterial genes in nature. This process requires competent cells, which are ready to accept extracellular plasmid and further stable replication inside recipient cells. Artificial transformation by preparing competent *E. coli* bacterial cells in lab is a common and widely used method in gene cloning. However, there are many naturally occurring competent bacteria, which participate in natural transformation like *Streptococcus pneumonia* and *Neisseria gonorrhoeae* [21]. Transformation constitutes a passive mode of plasmid invasion for otherwise non-mobile plasmids in niches that are rich in exogenous plasmid DNA (pDNA), for instance: aquatic environments [22] and biofilms. Free plasmid DNA is able to persist long enough to be available for uptake by competent bacteria *in situ* [23] (**Figures 1–3**).

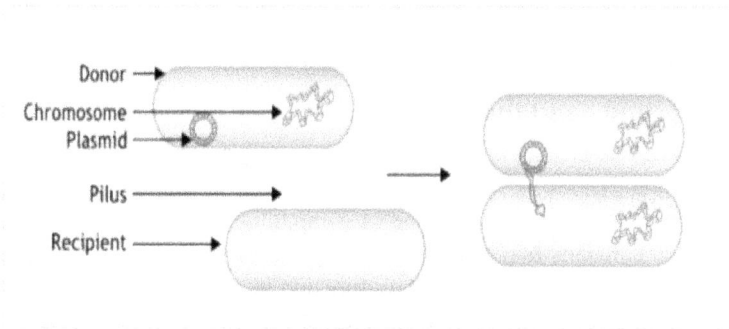

Figure 1. Transfer of plasmid between bacteria by conjugation [1].

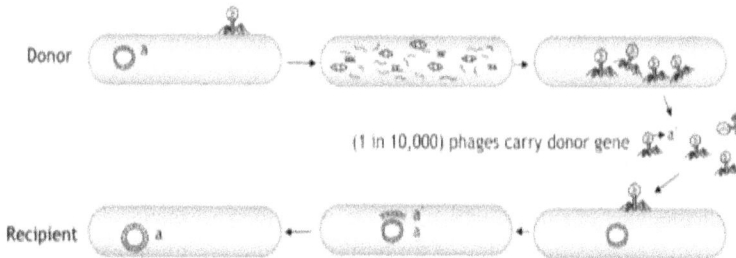

Figure 2. Gene transfer through transduction occurs between bacteriophages and bacteria [1].

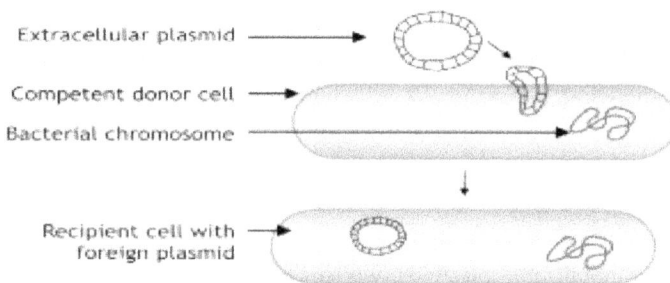

Figure 3. Extracellular plasmids are transferred to competent cells by the process of transformation [1].

7. Plasmid entry

Plasmid entrance into a host cell can be hindered at different levels, for instance: conjugative transfer of plasmids may be blocked by exclusion systems, which is responsible for maintaining plasmid exclusivity within a host [23]. Moreover, defense mechanisms against foreign DNA (example: restriction modification enzymes [24]) may act on plasmids during entrance. Co-hosting of the plasmids, which encode the related portioning systems may lead to interference during plasmid partition [25].

8. Types of plasmids and their functions

Plasmids are found in various bacteria, which are isolated from aquatic environments. When two different plasmids coexist, this is called as compatibility plasmid. When two plasmids are incompatible, this means that two plasmids are similar and are unable to coexist. Not only plasmids are classified according to their function in a host, but also they are classified according to their compatibility (depending on replication property) [8, 26–28].

There are five types of plasmids:

8.1. F-plasmid (fertility factor of *Escherichia coli* K-12)

Since it was the first plasmid to be described, scientists reported the occurrence of a peculiar infective inheritance mediated by an agent called F controlling the system of sex compatibility in *E. coli* K-12 strain [29, 30].

8.2. Col plasmid

A group of collicinogenic plasmids, which encode genes to synthesize colicins (bacteriocins). Such plasmids require DNA polymerase I for replication and are amplified by chloramphenicol (Cm) with the exception of ColE2. There are four groups of Col plasmids, which share a number of replication characteristics: CoL4, ColD, ColK, and ColEl [31].

8.3. R-plasmid

Some strains showed multiple resistant to six drugs as chloramphenicol (Cm), tetracycline (Tc), streptomycin (Sm), sulfisomidine (Su), ampicillin (Ap), and trimethoprim (Tp). Resistance property was co-transferred to *E. coli* by conjugation, which indicates that resistance was R plasmid-mediated [32].

8.4. Suicide plasmids

Such type of plasmids gets transferred to another bacterial cell but are not replicated further and are known as mobilizable plasmids, which are mostly used for transposon and gene replacement experiment [33].

8.5. Virulence plasmids

Presence of such plasmids increases pathogenicity of microbes. Different types of *E. coli* virulence plasmids exist, which are: enterotoxigenic *E. coli*, enteroinvasive *E. coli*, entero-pathogenic *E. coli*, enterohemorrahagic *E. coli*, enteroaggregative *E. coli*, and extraintestinal pathogenic *E. coli* [34].

9. Properties of plasmids

9.1. Heavy metal tolerance

Microbial method for heavy metal detoxification is widely used since it is highly specific for targeting heavy metal. General mechanisms involved in such kinds of tolerance are enzymatic alternation of the toxic compound, enzymatic modification of the target site, development of alternate metabolic pathways, and extrusion of the toxic compound from the cell [35]. Studies related to toxic metal ion tolerant bacteria increased rapidly after mercury-resistant bacteria (volatilize mercury) were discovered [36].

9.2. Nitrogen fixation

Nitrogen fixation in prokaryotic organisms is unique for having N_2 fixing ability as well as most of them is autotrophs. As in genes, N_2 fixing is conserved in chromosomal DNA and plasmids. Cyanobacteria are widely distributed and diverse group of autonomous bacteria, which mostly carry single or multiple phenotypically cryptic plasmids, for instance: analysis of unicellular *Cyanobacteria synechococcus* strains has revealed to carry homologous plasmids [37–40].

9.3. Sulfur utilization

A group of bacteria known as sulfur bacteria metabolize sulfur, which is useful for cycling sulfur in nature. Most of sulfur compounds, oxidized by Archaea and Bacteria are used as electron donors for anaerobic phototrophic and aerobic chemotrophic growth (oxidized to sulfate). The common energy sources for bacteria are hydrogen sulfide H_2S, sulfur and thio-sulfate S_2O_{32}. Scientists reported that oxidation of dibenzothiophene (DBT), which includes many sulfur-containing poly chromatic hydrocarbons is mediated by plasmid-borne functions in Pseudomonas isolates [41].

9.4. Hydrocarbon degradation

Hydrocarbon degradation is concerned mainly with environmental pollution and harmful impact. Such impacts of hydrocarbon pollution are oil spills, polyaromatic hydrocarbon pollution, which are absorbed to sediment and accumulated in aquatic animals like shellfish and fish followed by transfer to humans through seafood consumption [42]. Microbial degradation of hydrocarbons is a useful technique of bioremediation without any adverse impact on environment. Special genes are often carried on plasmids of bacteria [43]. Plasmids carrying structural genes for organic matter or xenobiotic degradation are called as degradative or catabolic plasmids. Experimentally proved, plasmids encoded the enzymes required for metabolizing naphthalene, salicylate, camphor, octane, xylene, and toluene [44]. Plasmid plays an essential role in polyaromatic hydrocarbon (PAH) degradation enhancing such capacity in the microbial community as in naphthalene degradation capacity [45].

9.5. Drug resistance

Multiple drug resistance is major issue since the early 1960s, when there were many reports concerning antibiotic resistance of Shigellae in south-east countries as Japan and Korea. In addition to that, drug resistance marked to be transferred other Enterobacteriaceae by conjugation. Resistance to antibiotics is acquired from factors called as R-factors, which are plasmids carrying resistant determinants (R-determinants) and resistance transfer factors (RTF). Anderson et al. reported that the two R-plasmid components are effective when found in the same cell. Since R-determinants are not transferable, RTF alone cannot develop drug resistance. Moreover, transfer of drug resistance depends on temperature and other physicochemical parameters of water, for instance: drug resistance of *Salmonella. typhi* isolated in Korea from 1968 to 1975 was more efficiently transferred to *E. coli* at 25°C than at 35°C. Most of drug resistance studies are aimed toward antibiotic resistance of human pathogenic bacteria such as Shigella and Salmonella. The antibiotics resistant to bacteria are; ampicillin (A), chloramphenicol (C), neomycin (N), kanamycin (K), streptomycin (S), sulfonamides (Su), and tetracycline (T) [46–48].

10. Uses of plasmids

Plasmids are utilized in biotechnology (most widely used for DNA manipulation, transfer, and gene expression in a variety of microorganisms and animal cells [49] and pharmaceutical biotechnology). In the latter field, plasmids are crucial in producing heterologous proteins, which substitute defective proteins present in the patient or provide a lost function due to lack of natural active protein. Since 1990s, transferring genes to humans was reported [50]. In addition to that, gene therapy and genetic vaccination have attracted more attention.

Gene therapy and DNA vaccination require the identification of gene(s) related to a particular disease (inherited/acquired), fabrication of therapeutic gene, the design of a molecular vector (and its formulation), and introduction of the gene into the patient. Once the gene is expressed in the patient, the correct patient is expected to be formed and function. However, problems related to recombinant protein production, for instance: complex glycosylation are eliminated. Possible related vectors exist to introduce genetic information into human cells. The most relevant are virus (adenovirus/retrovirus) and plasmid DNA (pDNA): both can be used in aqueous solution or included in lipids or other formulations.

Recently, over 1500 clinical trials of human gene therapy with more than 220 genes in almost 30 countries have been carried out since the first gene therapy trial was conducted: more than 60% of the trials have been performed in USA and around 30% in Europe. pDNA plays an essential role as a vector for gene therapy and DNA vaccination. Approximately, 20% of the trials for human gene therapy were based on naked pDNA, whereas lipofection (requiring pDNA production) counts for 6.6% of trials. Together, both approaches represent nearly 25% of techniques used in clinical trials [51].

11. Conclusion

Classifying plasmids by latest optical plasmid barcoding technology could be helpful in future advances in plasmid metagenomics, which intensifies the knowledge of plasmids through a range of environments and improves understanding of resistance gene reservoirs, thus leading to further investigations of plasmid biology. Viewing plasmid lifestyle transitions from the plasmid perspective opens up new branches for research on plasmid ecology and evolution. Also, plasmids are crucial for adaptation concerning genetic diversity. Plasmids possess properties related to xenobiotic degradation and heavy metal tolerance, which facilitates bioremediation of toxic chemicals in an eco-friendly manner. Concerning plasmid application, utilizing pDNA as a therapeutic agent has an important degree of efficacy demanding the development of better-produced strains, therefore, more efficient and scalable downstream processes are the need of day.

Conflict of interest

The authors declare that this chapter is written without any commercial or financial conflict of interest.

Author details

Munazza Gull* and Sondos El-Baz

*Address all correspondence to: munagull@hotmail.com

Biochemistry Department, Faculty of Science, King Abdulaziz University, Jeddah, Saudi Arabia

References

[1] Banu H, Prasad KP. Role of plasmids in microbiology. Journal of Aquaculture, Research and Development. 2017;8(1):1-8

[2] Frost LS, Koraimann G. Regulation of bacterial conjugation: Balancing opportunity with adversity. Future Microbiology. 2010;5(7):105-1071

[3]   Frost LS, Leplae R, Summers AO, Toussaint A. Mobile genetic elements: The agents of open source evolution. Nature Reviews. Microbiology. 2005;**3**:722

[4]   De Gelder L, Williams JJ, Ponciano JM, Sota M, Top EM. Adaptive plasmid evolution results in host-range expansion of a broad-host-range plasmid. Genetics. 2008; **178**(4):2179-2190

[5]   Hulter N, Ilhan J, Wein T, Kadibalban AS, Hammerschmidt K, Dagan T. An evolutionary perspective on plasmid lifestyle modes. Current Opinion in Microbiology. 2017;**38**:74-80

[6]   Orlek A, Stoesser N, Anjum MF, Michel D, Ellington MJ, Peto T, Crook D, Woodford N, Walker AS, Phan H, Sheppard AE. Plasmid classification in an era of whole-genome sequencing: Application in studies of antibiotic resistance epidemiology. Frontiers in Microbiology. 2017;**8**:1-10

[7]   Vivian A, Murillo J, Jackson RW. The roles of plasmids in phytopathogenic bacteria: Mobile arsenals? Microbiology. 2001;**147**(4):763-780

[8]   Shintani M, Sanchez ZK, Kimbara K. Genomics of microbial plasmids: Classification and identification based on replication and transfer systems and host taxonomy. Frontiers in Microbiology. 2015;**6**:1-16

[9]   Valverde A, Canton R, Garcillan-Barcia MP, Novais A, Galan JC, Alvarado A, de la Cruz F, Baquero F, Coque TM. Spread of blaCTX-M-14 is driven mainly by IncK plasmids disseminated among *Escherichia coli* phylogroups A, B1, and D in Spain. Antimicrobial Agents and Chemotherapy. 2009;**53**(12):5204-5212

[10] Garcillán-Barcia MP, Ruiz del Castillo B, Alvarado A, de la Cruz F, Martínez-Martínez L. Degenerate primer MOB typing of multiresistant clinical isolates of *E. coli* uncovers new plasmid backbones. Plasmid. 2015;**77**:17-27

[11] Carattoli A, Zankari E, García-Fernández A, Larsen MV, Lund O, Villa L, Møller AF, Hasman H. In silico detection and typing of plasmids using plasmidfinder and plasmid multilocus sequence typing. Antimicrobial Agents and Chemotherapy. 2014; **58**(7):3895-3903

[12] Villa L, García-Fernández A, Fortini D, Carattoli A. Replicon sequence typing of IncF plasmids carrying virulence and resistance determinants. Journal of Antimicrobial Chemotherapy. 2010;**65**(12):2518-2529

[13] Andreoni EF, Omiccioli E, Villa L, Magnani M, Carattoli A. Comparative analysis of the standard PCR-Based Replicon Typing (PBRT) with the commercial PBRT-KIT. Plasmid. 2017;**90**:10-14

[14] Carattoli A. Resistance plasmid families in *Enterobacteriaceae*. Antimicrobial Agents and Chemotherapy. 2009;**53**(6):2227-2238

[15] Carattoli A, Bertini A, Villa L, Falbo V, Hopkins KL, Threlfall EJ. Identification of plasmids by PCR-based replicon typing. Journal of Microbiological Methods. 2005;**63**(3):219-228

[16] Bertini A, Poirel L, Mugnier PD, Villa L, Nordmann P, Carattoli A. Characterization and PCR-based replicon typing of resistance plasmids in *Acinetobacter baumannii*. Antimicrobial Agents and Chemotherapy. 2010;**54**(10):4168-4177

[17] Jensen LB, Garcia-Migura L, Valenzuela AJS, Lohr M, Hasman H, Aarestrup FM. A classification system for plasmids from enterococci and other Gram-positive bacteria. Journal of Microbiological Methods. 2010;**80**(1):25-43

[18] Lozano C, García-Migura L, Aspiroz C, Zarazaga M, Torres C, Aarestrup FM. Expansion of a plasmid classification system for gram-positive bacteria and determination of the diversity of plasmids in *Staphylococcus aureus* strains of human, animal, and food origins. Applied and Environmental Microbiology. 2012;**78**(16):5948-5955

[19] Fulsundar S, Harms K, Flaten GE, Johnsen PJ, Chopade BA, Nielsen KM. Gene transfer potential of outer membrane vesicles of *Acinetobacter baylyi* and effects of stress on vesiculation. Applied and Environmental Microbiology. 2014;**80**(11):3469-3483

[20] Dubey GP, Ben-Yehuda S. Intercellular nanotubes mediate bacterial communication. Cell. 2011;**144**(4):590-600

[21] Lunsford RD. Streptococcal transformation: Essential features and applications of a natural gene exchange system. Plasmid. 1998;**39**(1):10-20

[22] Xue H, Cordero OX, Camas FM, Trimble W, Meyer F, Guglielmini J, Rocha EPC, Polza MF. Eco-evolutionary dynamics of episomes among ecologically cohesive bacterial populations. mBio. 2015;**6**(3):e00552-e00515

[23] Lorenze MG, Wackernagel W. Bacterial gene transfer by natural genetic transformation in the environment. Microbiology and Molecular Biology Reviews. 1994;**58**(3):563-602

[24] Sakuma T, Tazumi S, Furuya N, Komano T. ExcA proteins of IncI1 plasmid R64 and IncIγ plasmid R621a recognize different segments of their cognate TraY proteins in entry exclusion. Plasmid. 2013;**69**(2):138-145

[25] Hyland EM, Wallace EWJ, Murraya AW. A model for the evolution of biological specificity: A cross-reacting DNA-binding protein causes plasmid incompatibility. Journal of Bacteriology. 2014;**196**(16):3002-3011

[26] Solar del G, Giraldo R, Ruiz-Echevarría MJ, Espinosa M, Díaz-Orejas R. Replication and control of circular bacterial plasmids. Microbiology and Molecular Biology Reviews. 1998;**62**(2):434-464

[27] Maria PGB, Andrés A, de la, Fernando C. Identification of bacterial plasmids based on mobility and plasmid population biology. FEMS Microbiology Reviews. 2011;**35**:936-956

[28] Victoria FM, Athanasia V, Pilar G-BM, Amparo L, Constantin D, de la, Fernando C. A classification scheme for mobilization regions of bacterial plasmids. FEMS Microbiology Reviews. 2004;**28**:79-100

[29] Frost LS, Ippen-Ihler K, Skurray RA. Analysis of the sequence and gene products of the transfer region of the F sex factor. Microbiological Reviews. 1994;**58**(2):162-210

[30] Chris S, Pilar G-BM, Victoria FM, Rocha Eduardo PC, de la, Fernando C. Mobility of plasmids. Microbiology and Molecular Biology Reviews. 2010;**74**(3):434-452

[31] Johnson Timothy J, Nolan Lisa K. Pathogenomics of the virulence plasmids of *Escherichia coli*. Microbiology and Molecular Biology Reviews. 2009;**73**(4):750-774

[32] Riley Margaret A, Gordon David M. A survey of Col plasmids in natural isolates of *Escherichia coli* and an investigation into the stability of Col-plasmid lineages. Journal of General Microbiology. 1992;**138**:1345-1352

[33] Demarre G, Guérout A-M, Matsumoto-Mashimo C, Rowe-Magnus DA, Marlière P, Mazel D. A new family of mobilizable suicide plasmids based on broad host range R388 plasmid (IncW) and RP4 plasmid (IncPα) conjugative machineries and their cognate *Escherichia coli* host strains. Research in Microbiology. 2005;**156**(2):245-255

[34] Johnson J, Warren RL, Branstrom AA. Effects of FP2 and a mercury resistance plasmid from *Pseudomonas aeruginosa* PA103 on exoenzyme production. Journal of Clinical Microbiology. 1991;**29**(5):940-944

[35] Endo G, Ji G, Simon S. Heavy metal resistance plasmids and use in bioremediation. In: Moo-Young M et al., editors. Environmental Biotechnology: Principles and Applications. Netherland: Springer Netherlands; 1996. pp. 47-62

[36] Rasmussen LD, Zawadsky C, Binnerup SJ, Oregaard G, Sorensen SJ, Kroer N. Cultivation of hard-to-culture subsurface mercury-resistant bacteria and discovery of new mera gene sequences. Applied And Environmental Microbiology. 2008;**74**(12):3795-3803

[37] Ji G, Silver S. Bacterial resistance mechanisms for heavy metals of environmental concern. Journal of Industrial Microbiology. 1995;**14**(2):61-75

[38] Lebrun M, Audurier A, Cossart P. Plasmid-borne cadmium resistance genes in Listeria-monocytogenes are similar to Cada and Cadc of *Staphylococcus aureus* and are induced by cadmium. Journal of Bacteriology. 1994;**176**(10):3040-3048

[39] Berla BM, Saha R, Immethun CM, Maranas CD, Moon TS, Pakrasi HB. Synthetic biology of cyanobacteria: Unique challenges and opportunities. Frontiers in Microbiology. 2013;**4**(246):1-14

[40] Yang X, Mcfadden BA. A small plasmid, pCA2.4, from the Cyanobacterium *Synechocystis* sp. strain PCC 6803 encodes a rep protein and replicates by a rolling circle mechanism. Journal of Bacteriology. 1993;**175**(13):3981-3991

[41] Jensen AM, Finster KW, Karlson U. Degradation of carbazole, dibenzothiophene, and dibenzofuran at low temperature by *Pseudomonas* sp. strain C3211. Environmental Toxicology and Chemistry. 2003;**22**(4):730-735

[42] Meador JP, Stein JE, Reichert WL, Varanasi U. Bioaccumulation of polycyclic aromatic hydrocarbons by marine organisms. In: Ware GW, editor. Reviews of Environmental Contamination and Toxicology: Continuation of Residue Reviews. New York, NY: Springer; 1995. pp. 79-165

[43] Johnsen AR, Wick LY, Harms H. Principles of microbial PAH-degradation in soil. Environmental Pollution. 2005;**133**(1):71-84

[44] Leplae R, Lima-Mendez G, Toussaint A. A first global analysis of plasmid encoded proteins in the ACLAME database. FEMS Microbiology Reviews. 2006;**30**(6):980-994

[45] Foght JM, Westlake DWS. Transposon and spontaneous deletion mutants of plasmid-borne genes encoding polycyclic aromatic hydrocarbon degradation by a strain of *Pseudomonas fluorescens*. Biodegradation. 1996;**7**(4):353-366

[46] Anderson ES. Origin of transferable drug-resistance factors in the *enterobacteriaceae*. British Medical Journal. 1965;**2**(5473):1289-1291

[47] Chun D, Seol SY, Cho DT, Tak R. Drug resistance and R plasmids in *Salmonella typhi* isolated in Korea. Antimicrobial Agents and Chemotherapy. 1977;**11**(2):209-213

[48] Bennett PM. Plasmid encoded antibiotic resistance: Acquisition and transfer of antibiotic resistance genes in bacteria. British Journal of Pharmacology. 2008;**153**:S347-S357

[49] Palomares LA, Estrada-Moncada S, Ramírez OT. Production of recombinant proteins. In: Balbás P, Lorence A, editors. Recombinant Gene Expression: Reviews and Protocols. Totowa, NJ: Humana Press; 2004. pp. 15-51

[50] Rosenberg SA, Aebersold P, Cornetta K, Kasid A, Morgan RA, Moen R, Karson EM, Lotze MT, Yang JC, Topalian SL, Merino MJ, Culver K, Miller AD, Blaese RM, Anderson WF. Gene transfer into humans- immunotherapy of patients with advanced melanoma, using tumor-infiltrating lymphocytes modified by retroviral gene transduction. The New England Journal of Medicine. 1988;**323**(9):570-578

[51] Konishi M, Kawamoto K, Izumikawa M, Kuriyama H, Yamashita T. Gene transfer into Guinea pig cochlea using adeno-associated virus vectors. The Journal of Gene Medicine. 2008;**10**(6):610-618

Chapter 2

Plasmid Purification

Noboru Sasagawa

Additional information is available at the end of the chapter

http://dx.doi.org/10.5772/intechopen.76773

Abstract

Plasmid purification is a rather classical experiment, but the technique is still developing for time- and cost- saving. The critical principle is based on the alkaline lysis method, although the following steps have several variations. The needed purities and/or quantities of DNA depend on researches using isolated plasmids, meaning that more reasonable method can be selected in each experiment. For example, a non-alkaline-lysis method such as boiling method is still available. One of the important steps for purifying plasmid is a removal of RNA. Ribonuclease is usually used for removing RNA from plasmid sample. On the other hand, a kind of salts such as lithium and calcium functions to make RNA as a selective precipitate from DNA-RNA mixture. Based on these backgrounds, the technique to purify plasmid DNA has been discussed.

Keywords: plasmid DNA, chromosomal DNA, RNA, RNase, calcium, polyethylene glycol

1. Introduction

It is said that the word "plasmid" is first proposed by the Nobel Prize winner Joshua Lederberg [1, 2]. Plasmid is an extrachromosomal small circular deoxyribonucleic acid (DNA), which duplicates independently from chromosomal DNA. Although budding yeast and fission yeast can retain plasmid, the host of the plasmid is almost bacteria. This small circular DNA is widely used as DNA vector in molecular biology, biochemistry, biotechnology, cell biology, and so on. It means that plasmid purification/isolation is very fundamental experiment in these research fields, and that this experiment is achieved in almost every laboratories on almost every day.

2. A strategy for purifying plasmid from *Escherichia coli*

In biochemical aspects, to purify plasmid DNA from bacteria is to isolate only plasmid DNA from the mixture of biopolymers such as protein, ribonucleic acid (RNA), chromosomal DNA and plasmid DNA, by which bacteria cell is composed (**Figure 1**).

A chemical property of protein is totally different from nucleic acids; therefore, it is rather easy to separate nucleic acids and proteins. However, RNA and DNA are very similar molecules from each other. Among them, ribose in RNA is only distinguishable from deoxyribose in DNA by one hydroxyl group (–OH) at its structure. Furthermore, chromosomal DNA and plasmid DNA is both deoxyribonucleic acids that have the same chemical properties. Chromosomal DNA in almost all bacteria is circular, so is also plasmid. The distinguishable difference of them is only their size: plasmid DNA (~10 kilo base pairs) is much smaller than chromosomal DNA (4.6 million base pairs in *Escherichia coli*). Based on these properties, a special technique for purifying plasmid DNA among these biomolecules are required.

To purify plasmid DNA of high quantity, culture condition, or media for *E. coli* growth is also important [3].

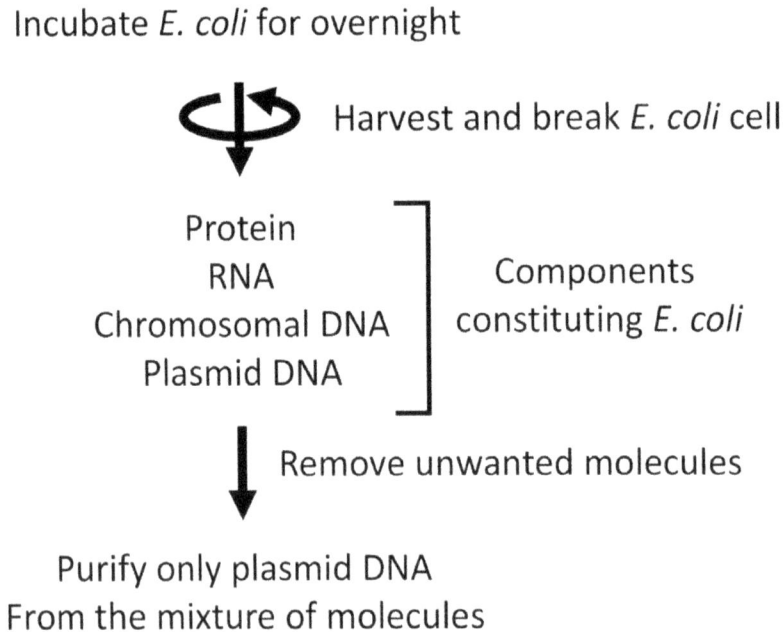

Figure 1. Strategy for purifying plasmid DNA from *E. coli*.

3. Very easy and simple way of plasmid preparation: boiling method

A very simple manipulation steps enable us to recover plasmid DNA from *Escherichia coli* (*E. coli*) (**Figure 2**) [4]. This experiment is called "Boiling method". In this experiment, STET solution (100 mM sodium chloride, 10 mM Tris-HCl (pH 8.0), 1 mM EDTA, 5% Triton-X or Tween 20) is added to *E. coli* pellet and suspended well. And then, the sample is heated to 100°C for 1 minute and centrifuged. After centrifugation, plasmid DNA is recovered in the solution, whereas insoluble heat-denatured proteins make debris as pellet fraction. After separating plasmid DNA from debris and precipitating plasmid DNA by adding alcohol, the final plasmid sample is capable for the next experiment, such as cutting plasmid by restriction enzyme and/or modifying DNA by other enzymes.

Interestingly, the pellet is rather moisty and easily removed by using toothpick and piercing it. This feature contributes to an easy handling of the experiment: we can achieve this plasmid extraction in only one tube from the start point to the end of the experiment. Therefore, boiling method has very convenient for handling many samples at a time. The modified boiling method, in which a concentrated STET solution is directly added to LB medium in which *E. coli* is grown, is also reported [5]. This modified method does not require even harvesting step of the grown bacteria by centrifugation.

The major disadvantage of the boiling method is that RNA is not removed in the principle of the boiling method and that the chromosomal DNA of *E. coli* is not completely removed from plasmid DNA. Therefore, the purity of the finally isolated plasmid DNA is not so high.

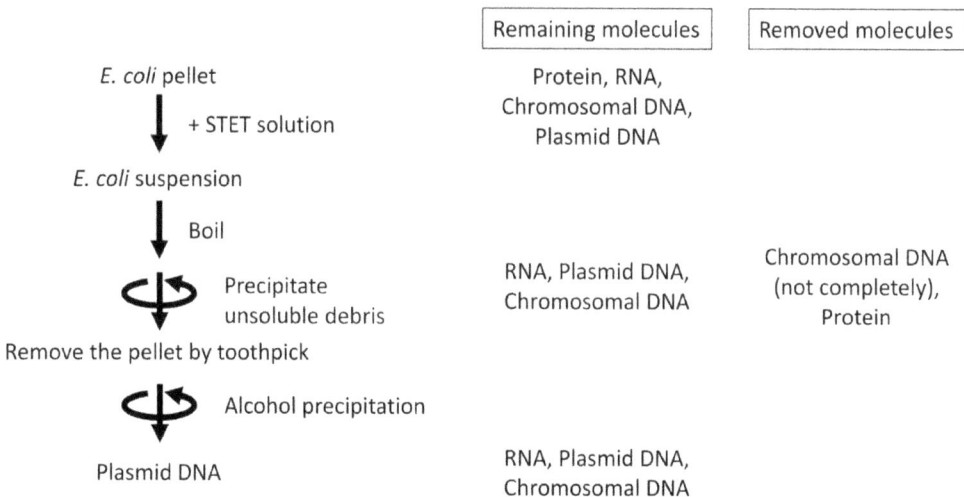

Figure 2. Scheme for purifying plasmid DNA by boiling method.

The boiling method is suitable for checking, if plasmid in *E. coli* transformant has an expected insert DNA (insert check), usually testing multiple samples at a time.

One substitution of the boiling method for insert check is colony polymerase chain reaction (PCR), directly adding *E. coli* colony to the PCR reaction mixture as a template. In colony PCR, *E. coli* cells are broken at the first 96°C step of PCR. Basically, a simple boiling of bacteria in the water is enough for collecting DNA from them, which has adequate quality to achieve PCR [6]. Colony PCR is much easier experiment than boiling method. However, once we isolate plasmid DNA even by rough purity of boiling method, we can further analyze the recovered plasmid by checking restriction enzyme patterns and so on. For example, restriction map is much informative result than if the fragment is amplified by colony PCR.

4. The definitive principle for plasmid isolation: denaturation of DNA double-strand by alkaline lysis

To purify plasmid from *E. coli*, there need each step for removing unnecessary molecules, such as protein, chromosomal DNA and RNA. For this purpose, alkaline denature of *E. coli* is the definitive technique for removing proteins and chromosomal DNA. This method was established in 1979 [7], but it is so sophisticated that almost all experiment for plasmid purification today is based on this technique (**Figure 3**).

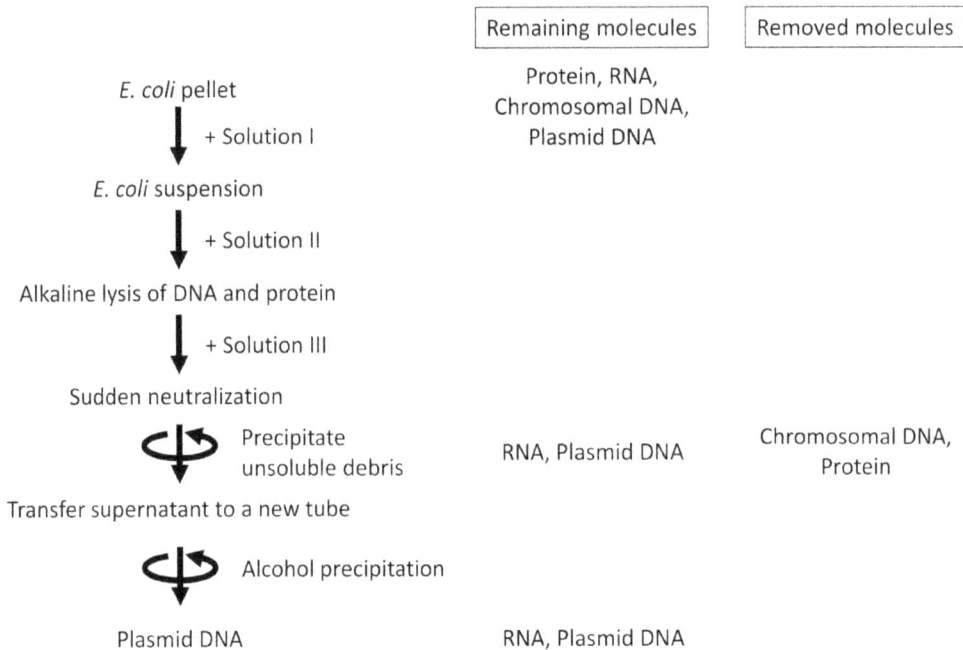

Figure 3. Scheme for alkaline lysis method.

The principle of the alkaline lysis method is a kind of magic. After suspending the *E. coli* in the solvent (solution I; 25 mM Tris/HCl (pH 8.0), 10 mM EDTA), an alkaline solution (solution II; 200 mM NaOH, 1% SDS) is added to the sample. In this condition, almost all proteins are denatured. DNA double-strand structure is also denatured to single-strand. However, even in such an extreme condition, supercoiled plasmid DNA remains its structure stable and not denatured. After 5 minutes, incubation of alkaline denature, high-salt buffer (solution III; 3 M Potassium Acetate, pH 5.5) is added for the purpose of a sudden change of pH in the solution. As a result, denatured protein and chromosomal DNA do not turn back to its own structure, causing these molecules insoluble. On the other hand, plasmid DNA remains soluble, thus centrifuge step easily separates the plasmid DNA from debris of proteins and chromosomal DNA. In the alkaline lysis method, each step is very simple and easy. All we have to do is only adding solution sequentially. Moreover, the function of each solution is only changing pH and salt concentration. However, these ingeniously planned three steps enable us to recover plasmid DNA, avoiding proteins and chromosomal DNA. The most notable point of this method is that we can isolate only plasmid DNA from plasmid/chromosomal DNA mixture; both are deoxyribonucleic acids and have the same chemical properties. No other method should successfully separate chromosomal DNA and plasmid DNA by such a simple step.

In early days, original protocol of alkaline lysis method used sodium acetate as a salt in solution III [7]. However, now potassium acetate is substituted for the major agent for solution III than sodium acetate. Potassium ion binds to dodecyl sulfate ion and forms potassium dodecyl sulfate (PDS). PDS is highly insoluble salt, which is made by adding solution III in the alkaline lysis sample. The PDS also plays a seed for insoluble debris, with which insoluble proteins and chromosomal DNA are co-precipitated. It is the great advantage that alkaline lysis method enables us to prevent protein and chromosomal DNA from plasmid at the same step.

One point we have to keep in mind is that supercoiled (closed circular) plasmid DNA is converted into nicked, relaxed (open circular) DNA by alkaline incubation. Thus, we have to keep the incubation time at solution II as in the instruction, and not to incubate the sample with solution II for a long time. Besides, RNA is not removed in a series of alkaline lysis method for plasmid purification (**Figure 3**). RNA is partially hydrolyzed by solution II but remains with the plasmid DNA at the final step. Therefore, a huge amount of RNA contamination is in the final plasmid DNA sample. Principally, only isolating plasmid DNA by alkaline lysis is inadequate for purifying high-quality plasmid DNA, and several schemes for further purification of the plasmid DNA, especially for removing RNA, should be needed.

Anyhow, alkaline lysis method has been the definitive way to initially purify the plasmid DNA.

5. RNA removal from plasmid sample

Neither alkaline lysis method nor boiling method does not isolate plasmid DNA from RNA mixture. An extra step for removing RNA is needed for further purification of plasmid DNA.

5.1. Ribonuclease (RNase)

Basically, to remove RNA (not to separate intact RNA) from DNA-RNA mixed solution is very easy: Only to add ribonuclease (RNase) to the solution enables us to completely digest RNA. Even when RNase is added to the solution I in the course of alkaline lysis method, RNA is completely digested in the finally corrected plasmid sample (see **Figure 3**). It sounds very strange that RNase in the solution I digest RNA, because the function of solution I is only to suspend the *E. coli*, the *E. coli* cell is not thought to lysed in the solution I step only. Otherwise, RNase might be still stable even in the alkaline condition of solution II, or rapidly renatured to the functional conformations in neutralized condition by solution III. RNase itself is a very stable protein, so we do not have to worry about a loss of enzyme activity at high-temperature. This character of RNase makes us very easy to handle this enzyme in the experiment, but this character often annoys us too, because a contamination of RNase to the other samples completely disturbs our RNA-handling experiment in the laboratory.

Irresponsible usage of RNase often contaminates the laboratory. Therefore, after incubating plasmid sample with RNase, the complete inactivation/removal of RNase should be needed.

5.2. Removal of RNase by phenol/chloroform extraction

Phenol or phenol/chloroform is well known as a protein denaturant. RNase is also inactivated by such as denaturant. Because RNase is very stable, repeating steps of phenol or phenol/chloroform extraction is effective for the complete removal of RNase. On the other hand, this organic reagent often inhibits enzyme activities, once contaminated with the nucleic acids samples. Besides, it is very convincing that phenol or phenol/chloroform have toxicity to cells, resulting in a decrease of transfection efficiency to cultured cells, and so on.

5.3. Salts as an agent for nucleic acid precipitation

It is known that a certain salts selectively precipitate nucleic acids. These salts can be applied to plasmid DNA purification.

5.3.1. Lithium chloride

Lithium chloride (LiCl) at the final concentration of 2.5 M enables us to selectively precipitate RNA. In this condition, RNA makes a pellet by centrifugation, but not DNA. Although low-molecular-weight RNA fragment is not precipitated and remains with plasmid DNA, it is often an adequate quality for using the plasmid in the following experiments, as long as the low-molecular-weight RNA makes critical disturbance for the experiment.

In isolating plasmid DNA by boiling method, Adding LiCl to STET is a better way to do the experiment (see **Figure 2**). After boiling step, centrifugation makes insoluble debris, together with RNA precipitation by the function of LiCl. Therefore, one-step centrifuge is enough for removing protein and RNA. Rather low-molecular-weight RNA still remains in the solution, but normally this RNA does not disturb or inhibit the activity of restriction enzyme and so on.

The insoluble pellet in the boiling method with LiCl is like a chewing gum, and is easily removed by picking with toothpick. Therefore, the combination of boiling method with LiCl is a very reasonable choice. One minor point is that LiCl is rather expensive than Calcium chloride ($CaCl_2$).

5.3.2. Calcium chloride

Calcium chloride ($CaCl_2$) is an inexpensive reagent. It is also known to precipitate RNA at the concentration of around 1 M, but DNA is not precipitated in this condition [8]. Thus, this reagent also works in the plasmid purification process like LiCl. However, it is a luck of luckiness that when $CaCl_2$ is added instead of LiCl in the boiling method, insoluble debris forms crumbly. This means that we cannot pick the debris up by using toothpick, and that we need another tube to transfer the supernatant after centrifugation. This disturbs a merit of the boiling method using only one tube all over the manipulations.

5.4. Polyethylene glycol precipitation of DNA

Polyethylene glycol (PEG) can be used to precipitate DNA [9]. It is also reported that the size of precipitated DNA is controllable by the concentration of PEG [10]. The principle of PEG precipitation is the same as alcohol precipitation, such us ethanol and/or isopropanol. This compound selectively precipitates DNA. Especially, low-molecular-weight RNA, such as transfer RNA, is not precipitated by PEG. There are so many products of PEG, according to their average molecular weights. Generally, PEG #3000, #4000, or #6000 has similar properties for DNA precipitation. Interestingly, to the contrast of that LiCl and $CaCl_2$ do not precipitate low-molecular-weight RNA, the size between precipitated RNA by salts and non-precipitated RNA by PEG precipitation are complementary in the RNA length from each other.

5.5. Cesium chloride ultracentrifuge

Cesium chloride (CsCl) ultracentrifuge method [11] does not require RNase. It means that phenol/chloroform extraction is not needed in the experiment, so plasmid DNA purified by this method is suitable for the almost all the biochemical experiment. That is, we can apply the plasmid DNA isolated by this method to transfection of the cultured cell and so on.

An ultrapure grade of plasmid is obtained in this method, although a special expensive ultracentrifuge is required for equipment. Moreover, very long time (almost overnight) for centrifuge is needed, and ethidium bromide (EtBr) at a very high concentration (final 800 μg/mL, this is 8000 times higher concentration than agarose gel electrophoresis) is used. EtBr is widely known as a mutagen, and highly concentrated EtBr should be unwanted to handle, if possible. EtBr intercalates to the double-strand of DNA. When this compound is intercalated with DNA, the double-strand of plasmid DNA changes to the slightly unwound form. This affects the sedimentation coefficient of nucleic acids in 10% CsCl solution. Therefore, supercoiled plasmid DNA makes a single sharp band in the tube after ultracentrifugation (200,000× *g*, 20°C, 16 hours). In this experiment, a specially customized tube should be used. The centrifuge tube is made of a soft, translucent plastic polymer, and the plasmid DNA is visualized as a band in the see-through tube. A syringe needle is inserted into the tube, and the separated plasmid band is sucked into the syringe. After transferring the sucked solution to a new tube, more extra steps are needed to get rid of CsCl and EtBr. This experiment is very sensitive to CsCl concentration. A slight change of CsCl amount causes a negative result; plasmid DNA is not separated as a single band in the tube.

CsCl ultracentrifuge method costs expensive because CsCl is an expensive reagent. Moreover, this experiment is time-consuming, hazardous, and difficult. On the contrary, once succeeded, we can obtain a large amount of ultrapure plasmid DNA. This method can even separate ccDNA from ocDNA, trusting the super high quality of plasmid DNA.

The important fact is that CsCl method is a kind of post-manipulation of alkaline lysis method. That is, alkaline lysis method is such a universal method that it works well as an initial step of CsCl method.

6. Standard plasmid purification method in recent days

Two major kit for plasmid purification is available in the market (**Figure 4**). Both use a basic alkaline lysis method for initial steps, and also uses RNase for RNA removal. A feature of the recent plasmid isolation methods is that they do not go through phenol/chloroform extraction after RNase treatment. Organic solvents are often harmful to cultured cell and so on, so avoiding this reagent in the steps of plasmid purification is a reasonable choice.

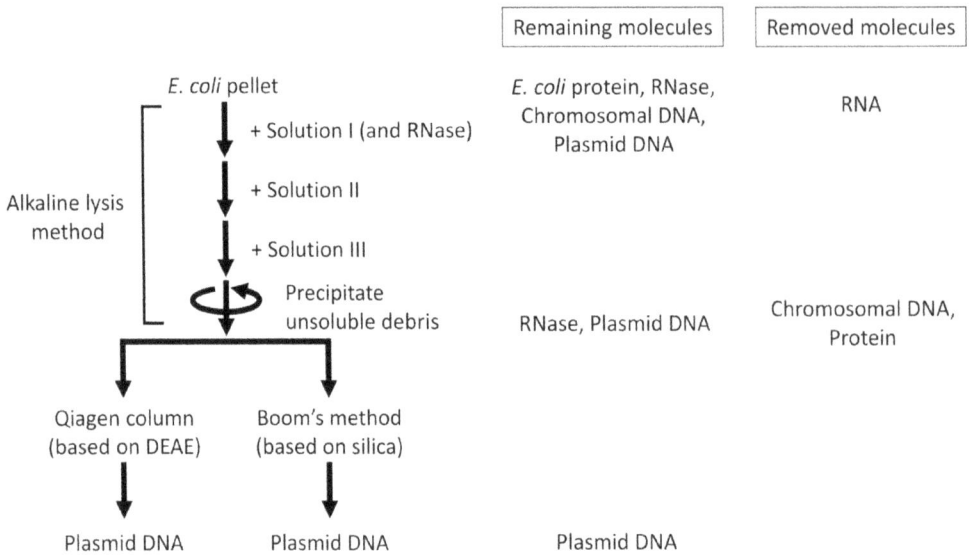

Figure 4. Qiagen kit and silica-membrane kit. They are widely used in many laboratories, but core principle is based on the definitive alkaline lysis method.

6.1. Qiagen column kit

Diethyl-aminoethyl (DEAE) group has positive charges; therefore DEAE-resin is often used to ion-exchange chromatography. DNA also has negative charges, so it binds to DEAE-resin under a certain pH or salt concentration. However, DNA purification by using DEAE was restricted to the recovery step from excised agarose gel and so on, because the binding property of nucleic acids to DEAE is rather broad and weak. Plasmid purification by anion-exchange chromatography has been reported [12], but it will be much better using the column as disposable to avoid contamination of samples. Therefore, DEAE was not seemed to be applicable for plasmid purification in a daily experiment. Qiagen column is famous for its ultrapure quality of purified plasmid DNA, and the principle is ion-exchange column chromatography. The precise information of Qiagen resin is confidential, but basically, it is known that the column consists of a highly condensed anion-exchange group resin [13]. In this experiment, the agent to remove RNA is not an ion-exchange resin, but RNase. A high concentration of RNase is added in the initial step of solution I. During Qiagen chromatography steps, the solutions go through a column in a free fall, so centrifuge step is not required at each step. However, after elution of the plasmid DNA from the resin, the concentration of plasmid DNA may be low, which is inadequate for the following experiment. Therefore, on Qiagen kit, ethanol precipitation is often needed to the eluted solution for concentrating plasmid. It seems that Qiagen columns are suitable for purifying plasmid of mini or maxi scale because the column is rather expensive. Besides, it is not easy to manipulate for multiple open columns at a time.

6.2. Boom's method (silica-membrane kit)

Boom's method is based on a paper and patent by Boom et al. [14], although the principle is widely known as a biochemical property of nucleic acids. The principle of Boom's method is that glass powder or diatomaceous earth (the main ingredient is SiO_2) adsorbs nucleic acids in a chaotropic condition [15], whereas proteins are not. In Boom's method, guanidine hydrochloride or guanidine thiocyanate is often used for chaotropic agent. This adsorption is reversibly eluted by pure water. Hydrophobic condition keeps the adsorption of DNA to SiO_2, so washing glass powder which adsorbs nucleic acids by 70% ethanol contributes to a high purity of plasmid DNA. The original Boom's method uses grass or diatomaceous earth powder as binding agent, and each step for binding, washing, and eluting is achieved as batch technique (simply centrifuging and discarding the solution). Batch chromatography is very simple method and easy to handle, although pipetting and discarding each solutions makes the experiment rather complicating for manipulating many samples at a time. On the other hand, the commercial kit supplies a column with a silica membrane filter, which is set to 1.5 mL microtube. Once the solution is applied to column, centrifuge step forces the solution go through the column. Therefore, each steps for binding, washing, and eluting needs only several seconds (as much as 1 minute) for centrifugation. Actually, commercial kit of such a silica membrane filter is very easy and useful for handling.

6.2.1. Homemade reagents for Boom's method

The commercial kit supplies their reagents with the column, but the compositions of these reagents are always confidential [16]. On the other hand, the principle of these kits seems almost the same, based on the DNA adsorption to silica matrix in chaotropic solution. Although it is quite natural to assume that each kit has its own special reagents, homemade solutions based on the original paper are generally available. When applied homemade reagents to commercial silica membrane column, quality and quantity of purified plasmid are almost the same as the commercial kit [17]. It means that these solutions are available by DIY and columns are not still waste, even when reagents in the commercial kit box are expired and out of use.

A modified reagent and modified protocol are also reported to increase the recovery efficiency of the plasmid DNA by commercial column [18]. On the other hand, not silica particles but Zirconium dioxide (ZrO_2, zirconia) has also been reported as an adsorbent of DNA [19].

6.2.2. Ultra-mini-scale purification

The chaotropic agent is a key factor in Boom's method, so guanidium salt such as GuHCl should play an important role for plasmid DNA purification in Boom's method. But it is reported that guanidium salt is not actually needed for nucleic acids to be adsorbed to silica particles. The other reagent such as high-concentration NaCl also works as chaotropic agent [20]. More surprisingly, a high concentration of the salt in solution III of alkaline lysis method seems already adequate for making the solution to chaotropic condition [21]. It means that adding guanidium for DNA adsorption can be skipped. To cut steps in the experiment has many advantages, especially for handling many samples at a time. Therefore, purifying plasmid samples in 96-well plate without guanidine chaotropic condition is proposed [21], in which method small scale and many samples at a time.

7. 55-minute method

Based on the alkaline lysis method, we developed a new plasmid purification method, which ends within 1 hour and does not need RNase (**Figure 5**) [22]. The principle of this method is a combination of the alkaline lysis method, $CaCl_2$ precipitation, and PEG precipitation. Although a sequential combination of these precipitations was already reported [23], our new invention is that we developed a new composition of solution III. This "super solution III" contains $CaCl_2$ to the standard solution III (Solution III: 5 M $CaCl_2$: H_2O = 2:2:1), which makes not only protein and genomic DNA debris but also a pellet of RNA in the debris. After centrifuging and recovering a supernatant, a standard PEG precipitation makes a plasmid DNA pellet and removes small RNA, which was not precipitated at the super solution III step. After all, only plasmid DNA remains in the final solution. Actually, this method needs totally 55 minutes from collecting *E. coli* pellet to recovering the final purified plasmid DNA. The great advantage of this method is that we are able to eliminate the use of RNase. Therefore, even RNase removal step is also eliminated. A quality and quantity are adequate for doing another experiment such as transfection into cultured cells.

	Remaining molecules	Removed molecules

E. coli pellet

Protein, RNA,
Chromosomal DNA,
Plasmid DNA

↓ + Solution I

E. coli suspension

↓ + Solution II

Alkaline lysis of DNA and protein

↓ + Super solution III

Sudden neutralization

Precipitate
unsoluble debris

Low-molecular weight RNA,
Plasmid DNA

Chromosomal DNA, Protein,
High-molecular weight RNA

Transfer supernatant to a new tube

PEG precipitation

Plasmid DNA

Plasmid DNA

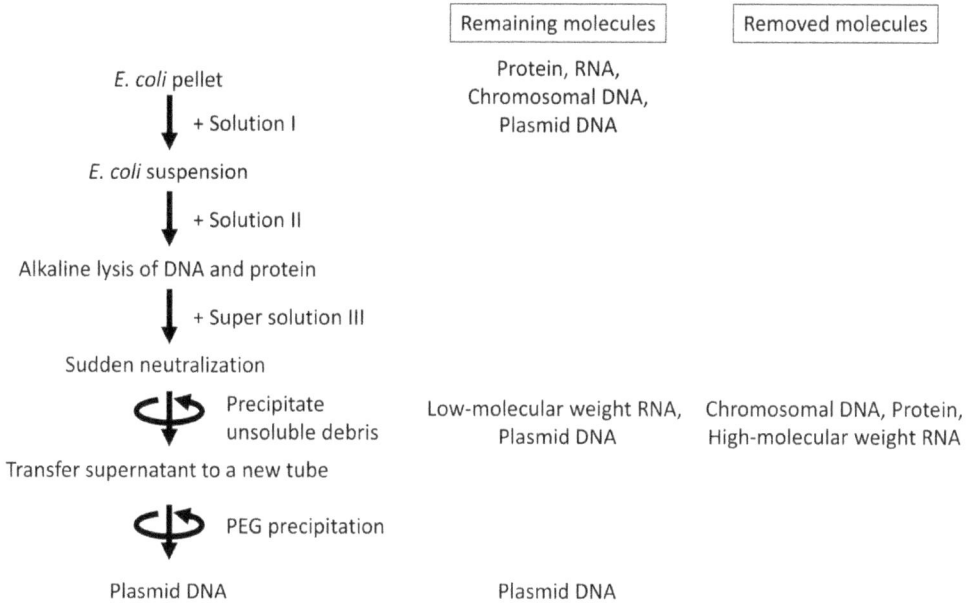

Figure 5. Scheme for 55 minutes method [17]. Note that it does not need to use RNase for RNA removal.

8. Conclusion

In a course of doing plasmid purification for every day, I noticed several tips for the experiment.

i. Alkaline denaturation/renaturation steps are so sophisticated that it is the definitive method for plasmid purification. None of another method will take over the alkaline lysis method. However, RNA is not removed in alkaline lysis method, so RNA removal steps should be applied in a course of plasmid isolation by alkaline lysis method.

ii. RNase is an easy choice to remove RNA, but should be completely removed after RNA digestion. One of the solutions is phenol/chloroform protein extraction, but phenol/chloroform may play a troublesome factor. Only a slight contamination of this reagent inhibits the activities of several enzymes and disturbs biochemical experiments. It also has toxicity to the cells, also disturbing transfection experiments. In other words, eliminating phenol/chloroform step in plasmid purification is the key point to trust its purity.

iii. Qiagen kits and Silica-membrane kits are actually the extra steps after alkaline lysis method. These kits need RNase for RNA digest. In other words, they work as RNase remover from the solution.

iv. RNase completely digests unwanted RNA from the plasmid sample. But this enzyme is very stable and very hard to inactivate, even disturbing RNA experiment in the laboratory.

Moreover, RNase is usually isolated from animals such as bovine, which may induce allergy to the human in gene therapy [24].

Based on these tips, we developed a new composition of solution III on alkaline lysis method, which enables us to purify plasmid DNA without adding of RNase. This method does not need any special columns or resins, but plasmid DNA purified by this method has enough quality for applying transfection to the cultured cell, injection into the nematode, and so on. Our result indicates that plasmid DNA purification without phenol/chloroform extraction is a great advantage for the quality of purified plasmid DNA.

Acknowledgements

I thank Ms. Haruka Yano (Tokai University Graduate School) for technical suggestions.

Conflict of interest

The author has no conflicts of interest directly relevant to the content of this article.

Notes/Thanks/Other declarations

The author has no other declarations about this article.

Author details

Noboru Sasagawa

Address all correspondence to: noboru.sasagawa@tokai-u.jp

Department of Applied Biochemistry, School of Engineering, Tokai University, Kanagawa, Japan

References

[1] Lederberg J. Cell genetics and hereditary symbiosis. Physiological Reviews. 1952;**32**: 403-430. DOI: 10.1152/physrev.1952.32.4.403

[2] Cohen SN. DNA cloning: A personal view after 40 years. Proceedings of the National Academy of Sciences of the United States of America. 2013;**110**:15521-15529. DOI: 10.1073/pnas.1313397110

[3]   Wood WN, Smith KD, Ream JA, Lewis LK. Enhancing yields of low and single copy number plasmid DNAs from *Escherichia coli* cells. Journal of Microbiological Methods. 2017;**133**:46-51. DOI: 10.1016/j.mimet.2016.12.016

[4]   Holmes DS, Quigley M. A rapid boiling method for the preparation of bacterial plasmids. Analytical Biochemistry. 1981;**114**:193-197

[5]   Elkin CJ, Richardson PM, Fourcade HM, Hammon NM, Pollard MJ, Predki PF, Glavina T, Hawkins TL. High-throughput plasmid purification for capillary sequencing. Genome Research. 2001;**11**:1269-1274. DOI: 10.1101/gr.167801

[6]   Peng X, Yu KQ, Deng GH, Jiang YX, Wang Y, Zhang GX, Zhou HW. Comparison of direct boiling method with commercial kits for extracting fecal microbiome DNA by Illumina sequencing of 16S rRNA tags. Journal of Microbiological Methods. 2013;**95**: 455-462. DOI: 10.1016/j.mimet.2013.07.015

[7]   Birnboim HC, Doly J. A rapid alkaline extraction procedure for screening recombinant plasmid DNA. Nucleic Acids Research. 1979;**7**:1513-1523

[8]   Eon-Duval A, Gumbs K, Ellett C. Precipitation of RNA impurities with high salt in a plasmid DNA purification process: Use of experimental design to determine reaction conditions. Biotechnology and Bioengineering. 2003;**83**:544-553. DOI: 10.1002/bit.10704

[9]   Paithankar KR, Prasad KS. Precipitation of DNA by polyethylene glycol and ethanol. Nucleic Acids Research. 1991;**19**:1346

[10] Hartley JL, Bowen H. PEG precipitation for selective removal of small DNA fragments. Focus. 1996;**18**:27

[11] Green MR, Sambrook J. Preparation of plasmid dna by alkaline lysis with sodium dodecyl sulfate: Maxipreps. Cold Spring Harbor Protocols. 2018. DOI: 10.1101/pdb.prot093351

[12] Grunwald AG, Shields MS. Plasmid purification using membrane-based anion-exchange chromatography. Analytical Biochemistry. 2001;**296**:138-141. DOI: 10.1006/abio.2001.5197

[13] QIAGEN Plasmid Purification Handbook. 2nd ed. QIAGEN; 2003. pp. 76-77

[14] Boom R, Sol CJ, Salimans MM, Jansen CL, Wertheimvan Dillen PM, van der Noordaa J. Rapid and simple method for purification of nucleic acids. Journal of Clinical Microbiology. 1990;**28**:495-503

[15] Marko MA, Chipperfield R, Birnboim HC. A procedure for the large scale isolation of highly purified plasmid DNA using alkaline extraction and binding to glass powder. Analytical Biochemistry. 1982;**121**:382-387

[16] GenElute™ Plasmid Miniprep Kit. Sigma-Aldrich; 2010

[17] Sasagawa N, Yano H. Plasmid DNA Purification using specialized reagents. Proceedings of the School of Engineering of Tokai University. 2017;**57**:1-4

[18] Pronobis MI, Deuitch N, Peifer M. The Miraprep: A protocol that uses a Miniprep kit and provides Maxiprep yields. PLoS One. 2016;**11**:e0160509. DOI: 10.1371/journal. pone.0160509

[19] Saraji M, Yousefi S, Talebi M. Plasmid DNA purification by zirconia magnetic nanocomposite. Analytical Biochemistry. 2017;**539**:33-38. DOI: 10.1016/j.ab.2017.10.004

[20] Lakshmi R, Baskar V, Ranga U. Extraction of superiorquality plasmid DNA by a combination of modified alkaline lysis and silica matrix. Analytical Biochemistry. 1999;**272**: 109-112. DOI: 10.1006/abio.1999.4125

[21] Neudecker F, Grimm S. High-throughput method for isolating plasmid DNA with reduced lipopolysaccharide content. BioTechniques. 2000;**28**:106-108

[22] Sasagawa N, Koebis M, Yonemura Y, Mitsuhashi H, Ishiura S. A high-salinity solution with calcium chloride enables RNase-free, easy plasmid isolation within 55 minutes. BioScience Trends. 2013;**7**:270-275

[23] Sauer ML, Kollars B, Geraets R, Sutton F. Sequential $CaCl_2$, polyethylene glycol precipitation for RNase-free plasmid DNA isolation. Analytical Biochemistry. 2008;**380**:310-314. DOI: 10.1016/j.ab.2008.05.044

[24] Eon-Duval A, MacDuff RH, Fisher CA, Harris MJ, Brook C. Removal of RNA impurities by tangential flow filtration in an RNase-free plasmid DNA purification process. Analytical Biochemistry. 2003;**316**:66-73

Plasmids Current Research and Future Trends

Chapter 3

Plasmids for Optimizing Expression of Recombinant Proteins in *E. coli*

Ahmed Mahmoud Al-Hejin, Roop Singh Bora and
Mohamed Morsi M. Ahmed

Additional information is available at the end of the chapter

http://dx.doi.org/10.5772/intechopen.82205

Abstract

Plasmids are important vectors for the transfer of genetic material among microbes. The transfer of plasmids causes transmission of genes involved in pathogenesis and survival, to the host bacteria leading to their evolution and adaptation to diverse environmental conditions. A large number of plasmids of varying sizes have been discovered and isolated from various microorganisms. Plasmids are also valuable tools to genetically manipulate microbes for various purposes including production of recombinant proteins. *Escherichia coli* is the most preferred microbe for production of recombinant proteins, due to rapid growth rate, cost-effectiveness, high yield of the recombinant proteins and easy scale-up process. Several plasmids have been designed to optimize the expression of heterologous proteins in *E. coli*. In order to circumvent the issues of protein refolding, the codon usage in *E. coli*, the absence of post-translational modifications, such as glycosylation and low recovery of functionally active recombinant proteins, various plasmids have been designed and constructed. This chapter summarizes the recent technological advancements that have extended the use of the *E. coli* expression system to produce more complex proteins, including glycosylated recombinant proteins and therapeutic antibodies.

Keywords: plasmid, recombinant protein, promoter, codon usage, molecular chaperones, fusion tags

1. Introduction

Plasmids are defined as extrachromosomal double-stranded circular DNAs within a cell that have the capability to replicate independently of chromosomal DNA. Plasmids are found in many microorganisms including bacteria, archaea and some eukaryotes such as yeast [1].

The advent of new DNA sequencing technologies has successfully determined the complete sequence of 4602 plasmids; most of these plasmids, that is, 4418 are from bacteria, 137 plasmids are identified from archaea and 47 plasmids are identified from eukaryotes [2]. The size of plasmids can vary between 1 and 200 kb, and they more often harbour genes encoding proteins that confer selective advantage to host cells under adverse conditions. Some of the genes are known as resistance genes which confer resistance to certain antibiotics. Genes involved in synthesis of antibiotics and various kinds of toxins are also localized on plasmids. Some of the genes present on plasmids encode for various virulence factors that assist microbes to colonize host and escape from its defence mechanisms. Plasmids also harbour genes that empower bacteria to fix nitrogen.

Plasmids can be present in a single bacterial cell in varying number which may range from one to few hundreds. The usual number of plasmids that are present in an individual cell is termed as copy number and is governed by the size of plasmid and the regulation of replication initiation. Large-size plasmids are present in low copy number and exist as one or very few copies in single bacterium. Such single-copy plasmids employ parABS and parMRC systems, termed as partition system, to equally segregate a copy of plasmid to each daughter cell upon cell division [3].

Independent replication of plasmids requires the presence of a region of DNA that can serve as an origin of replication. A self-replicating unit is termed as a replicon. A classical bacterial replicon comprises of gene for plasmid-specific replication initiation protein (Rep), DnaA boxes, AT-rich region and repeating units called iterons [4]. Large-size plasmids also harbour genes required for their replication, while smaller plasmids employ host replicative machinery to undergo replication.

Plasmids can be transmitted from one bacteria to another by the process of conjugation, and it has been reported that approximately 14% of the currently known plasmids are conjugative [5, 6]. Conjugation is a very efficient mechanism to transfer genes among microbes and thus facilitate the rapid evolution and adaptation of microbes to various adverse environmental conditions [7]. This transfer of genes among bacteria is one mechanism of horizontal gene transfer and is responsible for spread of antibiotic resistance among pathogenic microbes [8, 9].

Plasmids are very commonly used as vectors in the field of genetic engineering for the purpose of cloning and expression of desired genes. Various types of plasmids are now available commercially for cloning and expression of foreign genes in a wide variety of host including *E. coli*, yeast and mammalian cells [10]. The desired genes to be cloned and expressed are inserted into suitable plasmid. For cloning purpose, plasmid vectors are designed to contain a site, known as multiple cloning site (MCS) or polylinker site, which allows insertion of heterologous genes. The multiple cloning site contains several commonly used restriction sites for Type III restriction enzymes. The plasmid vectors contain an origin of replication, which allows its replication in bacterial host. Besides, these plasmids also harbour a gene that confers resistance to a specific antibiotic such as ampicillin or kanamycin which is used as a selectable marker. After the insertion of desired heterologous gene into multiple cloning site of the plasmid vector, the constructed plasmid is introduced into bacterial cells by the process of transformation. The transformed cells are further exposed to selective growth medium containing the specific antibiotic. The cells that contain the introduced plasmid will be able to survive and grow in selective medium as they carry the plasmid with the antibiotic resistance gene. This strategy is employed to clone and express heterologous proteins in *E. coli* for the large-scale production of recombinant proteins for therapeutics and wide variety of functional studies [10]. In this chapter, we summarize the recent technological advancements in the field of molecular biology that have extended the use of the *E. coli* expression system to produce more complex proteins, including glycosylated recombinant proteins and therapeutic antibodies.

2. *E. coli* as an expression system for production of recombinant proteins

Escherichia coli is a very commonly used, robust and cost-effective expression system for large-scale production of recombinant proteins. *E. coli* is genetically well characterized and is easy to handle and manipulate genetically. Its faster growth rate, inexpensive culture media, high expression levels and easy scale-up process provide major advantages for large-scale production of recombinant proteins for therapeutic purposes or various functional studies [11]. *E. coli* was successfully used to manufacture recombinant human insulin in 1982 for treating diabetes patients. It is important to note that insulin is a heterodimer and entails oxidative protein folding to attain a functionally active 3D conformation. The success accomplished with high level expression of recombinant human insulin validated the significance of *E. coli* expression system for large-scale production of recombinant proteins. Besides human insulin, several recombinant proteins for therapeutic applications, including human growth hormone, interferon α2a and α2b, glucagon, urate oxidase, granulocyte colony-stimulating factor and parathyroid hormone, have been successfully manufactured using *E. coli* expression system [12]. Although *E. coli* has been used extensively for expression of heterologous proteins, it is still not possible to determine the optimum production conditions for all the proteins. Expression conditions that are optimal for one protein may not be ideal for another protein. One of the major issues while producing heterologous proteins in *E. coli* is differences in codon usage between the two organisms. This difference in codon usage could cause errors in translation leading to low expression levels of recombinant proteins [13]. The other parameters that can affect the protein expression are choice of promoters, growth conditions and hydrophobicity of proteins.

3. Promoter

Promoter is a very critical region in plasmid vectors, used for the expression of heterologous proteins. Promoter is a stretch of DNA that is involved in the initiation of transcription of a gene and is located upstream of the transcription initiation site of gene. Promoters are normally 100–1000 base pairs in size. In *E. coli* and other bacterial species, promoter encompasses two short DNA sequences that are 10 nucleotides (termed as the Pribnow Box) and

35 nucleotides upstream from the transcription initiation site. The consensus sequence at −10 region is 'TATAAT' and the consensus sequence at −35 region is 'TTGACA'. This promoter sequence is recognized by RNA polymerase which leads to initiation of transcription. Several plasmids with strong or weak promoter are now available to express heterologous proteins in *E. coli*. Some of the commonly used promoters in *E. coli* expression vectors include T7 promoter, derived from bacteriophage T7, *E. coli* lac promoter, its improved modified version lacUV5 and Tac promoter produced from the combination of trp and lac promoters (**Table 1**). Another important promoter is the trc promoter, which is originated from lacUV5 and trp promoters. The potency of a promoter is governed by the frequency of transcription initiation which is regulated by the affinity of RNA polymerase for the promoter sequence. The T7 promoter is very strong as compared to *E. coli* promoters due to high frequency of transcription initiation and efficient processivity and hence it is routinely used for very high expression

Plasmid	Promoter	Origin of replication	Antibiotic selection marker	Fusion tags	Size of the fusion tag	Protease cleavage site	Vendor
pGEX-2 T	tac	pBR322	Ampicillin	GST	26 kDa	Thr	Pharmacia
pGEX-3X	tac	pBR322	Ampicillin	GST	26 kDa	Xa	Pharmacia
pGEX-6P	tac	pBR322	Ampicillin	GST	26 kDa	Pre	Pharmacia
pMAL-c2X	tac	ColE1	Ampicillin	MBP	42 kDa	Xa	New England Biolabs
pMAL-c2E	tac	ColE1	Ampicillin	MBP	42 kDa	EK	New England Biolabs
pQE-30/31/32	T5-lac	ColE1	Ampicillin	N-6XHis	1 kDa	None	Qiagen
pTrxFus	PL	ColE1	Ampicillin	TRX	11.6 kDa	EK	Invitrogen
pET-14b	T7	pBR322	Ampicillin	N-6XHis	1 kDa	Thr	Novagen
pET-19b	T7-lac	pBR322	Ampicillin	N-6XHis	1 kDa	EK	Novagen
pET-29a-c(+)	T7-lac	pBR322	Kanamycin	C-6XHis	1 kDa	Thr	Novagen
pET-41a-c(+)	T7-lac	pBR322	Kanamycin	GST	26 kDa	Thr	Novagen
pET-43a-c(+)	T7-lac	pBR322	Kanamycin	NusA	55 kDa	Thr	Novagen
pET-SUMO	T7	pBR322	Kanamycin	SUMO	11 kDa	SUMO protease	Invitrogen

GST, Glutathione S-transferase; MBP, maltose-binding protein; TRX, thioredoxin; NusA, N-Utilization substance A; N-6XHis, N-terminus 6X-histidine; C-6XHis, C-terminus 6X-histidine; SUMO, small ubiquitin-like modifier (SUMO); Thr, Thrombin; Xa, Factor Xa; Pre, PreScission; EK, Enterokinase;

Source: http://wolfson.huji.ac.il/expression/bac-strains-prot-exp; http://www.emdmillipore.com/life-science-research/novagen; http://www.invitrogen.com/1/3/stratagene-products https://www.neb.com

Table 1. List of some commonly used plasmids for improving expression levels and solubility of recombinant proteins in *E. coli*.

levels of recombinant proteins. However, in some instances, large-scale production of recombinant proteins can lead to its accumulation as insoluble aggregates also known as inclusion bodies, which can cause poor yield of biologically active recombinant proteins. In such cases, the use of expression vector containing a weak promoter such as the trc promoter instead of the T7 promoter can enhance protein solubility [14].

4. Ribosomal binding site

Ribosomal binding site is a very crucial component in plasmids commonly used for expression of recombinant proteins in *E. coli*. It is comprised of translation initiation codon, that is, AUG and the Shine-Dalgarno (SD) sequence and is required for efficient translation initiation [15]. Shine-Dalgarno sequence is localized 7–9 nucleotides upstream from the initiation codon and the consensus SD sequence is AAGGAGG. Various factors are known to affect translation initiation such as secondary structure of ribosomal binding site, consensus SD sequence, varying number of thymine and adenine and also the nucleotides upstream and downstream of the initiation codon AUG [16]. The translation efficiency is enhanced by the presence of more number of adenine and thymine in the ribosomal binding site. Highly expressed genes are found to contain adenine after the initiation codon [17]. Park and colleagues designed various variants of 5′-untranslated region (UTR) comprising of SD sequence and the AU-rich region, using PCR-based site-directed mutagenesis and analysed their impact on protein expression levels [18]. Such a strategy of modifying 5′UTR could be of immense value to improve translation efficiency and obtain high expression level of recombinant proteins. Incorporation of simple variations in 5′UTR could be exploited to optimize the expression of heterologous proteins [18, 19]. Another important factor that could affect the translation efficiency is the secondary structures in mRNA which could lead to variations in protein expression levels. The RNA helicase DEAD protein of *E. coli* can be exploited to remove secondary structures in mRNA. It had been demonstrated that co-expression of DEAD protein increased the expression of β-galactosidase from T7 promoter by several fold, implying that DEAD-box protein is involved in stabilizing the mRNA [20, 21]. This property of DEAD-box protein can be used to enhance the expression of genes which are poorly expressed due to secondary structures of mRNA. Protein translation is a highly efficient process as any error during translation could cause mutations, misincorporation of amino acids and low expression levels and hence can severely affect the quality of recombinant proteins produced in *E. coli*.

5. Codon usage and plasmid containing tRNA genes cognate to the rare codons

Codon usage is a major issue while expressing heterologous proteins, particularly human proteins in *E. coli*. There are marked differences in codon usage between *E. coli* and humans. Codons that are found to be very common in human and other eukaryotic genes are very rare in *E. coli*. Presence of rare codons in heterologous genes can lead to errors in translation and cause low expression levels of recombinant protein in *E. coli*. The presence of rare codons in heterologous genes might cause translational errors due to ribosomal stalling at these positions. These translational errors include frame-shift mutations, amino acid substitutions or premature translation termination [22]. Some of the rare codons in *E. coli* that cause problems in recombinant proteins are AGA, CGG, CGA, AGG (arginine), AAG (lysine), GGA (glycine), CUA (leucine), AUA (isoleucine) and CCC (proline) [23]. In *E. coli,* CGG is a rare arginine codon which occurs at a frequency of 0.54%. McNulty and colleagues demonstrated that the presence of large number of rare arginine codon CGG in p27 protease domain from Herpes Simplex Virus 2 (HSV- 2) resulted in the synthesis of recombinant protein of molecular weight that was 3 kDa higher than the actual molecular weight when expressed in *E. coli* [22]. The resultant increase in molecular weight was found to be due to the +1 frame-shift mutation at one of the CGG codons at the C-terminus of the viral protein. Besides, glutamine residues were misincorporated instead of arginine due to misreading of CGG as CAG [22].

Various strategies have been designed to circumvent the problem of codon bias in *E. coli* for enhancing the production of authentic, biologically active heterologous recombinant proteins. One strategy is to synthesize the full-length gene based on codon usage, but the high cost of gene synthesis is a major drawback. Another strategy requires site-directed mutagenesis of the foreign gene to generate codons which correlates with the tRNA pool of *E. coli*. However, this process is very expensive and time-consuming. Another approach is to co-transform the *E. coli* with plasmid containing the tRNA gene cognate to the rare codons. By increasing the copy number of rare tRNA genes, *E. coli* strains can be designed to complement the codon usage frequency in the foreign gene. This strategy is very feasible and cost-effective and highly efficient for expression of heterologous genes harbouring large number of rare codons. McNulty and colleagues carried out the co-expression of argX gene which codes for the cognate tRNA for rare arginine codon CGG, with the p27 protease domain of HSV-2 in order to circumvent the problem of codon bias. It was observed that the co-expression of cognate tRNA gene for CGG codon resulted in abolition of both frame-shift mutation and glutamine misincorporation and enhanced the expression levels of authentic recombinant protein by up to sevenfold [22]. This study clearly suggested that supplementation of the cognate tRNA for the rare codons such as CGG can alleviate the CGG codon bias in *E. coli* and hence lead to accurate and efficient synthesis of recombinant proteins. This strategy is now routinely being employed for several difficult-to-express heterologous recombinant proteins containing rare codons, in *E. coli*. Currently, several plasmids such as pRARE plasmids are commercially available which harbour genes encoding for tRNA cognate to rare codons. Another important feature in these pRARE plasmids is the presence of p15A replication origin, which facilitate their maintenance in the presence of compatible ColE1 origin of replication, commonly present in several *E. coli* expression vectors. Moreover, several *E. coli* strains are now commercially available that carry plasmids containing tRNA genes for cognate rare codons, such as BL21(DE3) CodonPlus-RIL and Rosetta (DE3). Tegel and colleagues analysed the expression of several human proteins in *E. coli* strain Rosetta (DE3) harbouring pRARE plasmid and observed that the total yields of the 35 recombinant proteins out of 68 proteins tested were enhanced significantly [24].

6. Plasmids carrying molecular chaperones for optimization of protein folding

Production of recombinant proteins for therapeutic purposes or various functional studies requires a robust and cost-effective expression system which can synthesize heterologous proteins in soluble form. Although *E. coli* expression system is always a preferred choice for expression of recombinant proteins, accumulation of foreign proteins as insoluble aggregates, also called as inclusion bodies, is a major problem. Recovery of proteins from these inclusion bodies is a very cumbersome process which entails denaturation and renaturation steps to obtain recombinant protein in properly folded and soluble form. However, this extraction process causes tremendous loss of proteins and further reduces the total yield of biologically active recombinant proteins. One approach to enhance the solubility of heterologous protein and reduce the formation of inclusion bodies is to employ molecular chaperones. It is now known that molecular chaperones assist the nascent polypeptide to fold properly during the process of protein synthesis and thus prevent protein aggregation. Few molecular chaperones are found to improve folding and solubilization of misfolded protein, while other chaperones are involved in prevention of protein aggregation [25–27]. The commonly used molecular chaperones in *E. coli* are GroEL, GroES, DnaK, DnaJ and Trigger factor (**Table 2**). These cytoplasmic chaperones can be employed either individually or in combination of different chaperones to enhance protein solubility and prevent formation of inclusion bodies [10, 26, 28, 29]. The GroEL-GroES chaperone combination is highly efficient to enhance protein refolding and also prevent protein degradation. It has been shown that Trigger factor interacts with GroEL and increases GroEL-substrate binding to improve protein folding [30]. Some chaperones such as heat shock proteins IpbA and IpbB prevent aggregation of heat denatured proteins [31]. It is advisable to test different combinations of molecular chaperones to identify the most efficient combination for improving the solubility of heterologous recombinant proteins. Co-expression of molecular chaperones Skp and FkpA in *E. coli* had been shown to improve the solubility of antibody fragments [32]. Combination of GroEL-GroES chaperones was found to be very efficient in production of anti-B-type natriuretic peptide single-chain antibody (scFv), as 65% of the expressed protein was in soluble form, which was almost 2.4-fold more than the one obtained in the absence of chaperones [33].

Plasmid	Chaperones	Promoter	Antibiotic marker	Inducer	Vendor
pGro7	*gro*ES-*gro*EL	*araB*	Chloramphenicol	L-Arabinose	TaKaRa
pKJE7	*dna*K-*dna*J-*grp*E	*araB*	Chloramphenicol	L-Arabinose	TaKaRa
pG-KJE8	*dna*K-*dna*J-*grp*E *gro*ES-*gro*EL	*araB Pzt-1*	Chloramphenicol	L-Arabinose Tetracycline	TaKaRa
pTf16	Trigger factor (tig)	*araB*	Chloramphenicol	L-Arabinose	TaKaRa
pG-Tf2	*gro*ES-*gro*EL-tig	*Pzt-1*	Chloramphenicol	Tetracycline	TaKaRa
pBB540	grpE, clpB	Lac	Chloramphenicol	IPTG	Addgene

Table 2. List of plasmids carrying molecular chaperones for improving protein folding in *E. coli*.

It has been demonstrated that the periplasm of *E. coli* presents an ideal environment to express complex therapeutic proteins including antibody fragments. The oxidizing condition and Dsb protein family in the periplasm provide ideal environment for proper disulphide bond formation and folding of recombinant proteins. Moreover, very few host proteins are present in the periplasm, which leads to high yield of purified recombinant proteins. Therapeutic antibodies such as Lucentis and Cimzia (Fab fragments) and few full-length aglycosylated antibodies and scFvs have been successfully produced by periplasmic expression in *E. coli* [34, 35]. Yim and colleagues employed the endoxylanase signal peptide to produce large amount of granulocyte colony-stimulating factor (GCSF) at 4.2 g/l in the periplasm of *E. coli* [36]. Co-expression of periplasmic chaperones can be exploited to improve the expression of properly folded protein in periplasm of *E. coli*. Overexpression of periplasmic chaperones DsbA and DsbC was found to enhance the efficiency of the assembly of the heavy chain and light chain of antibody in the periplasm of *E. coli* and drastically increased the production of full-length antibody from 0.1 to 1.05 g/l [37]. Co-expression of anti-CD20 scFv antibody with the periplasmic chaperone Skp resulted in the enhanced yield as well as antigen binding of antibody [38]. Lee and colleagues developed a highly efficient *E. coli* expression system to produce full-length antibody, by modifying 5′UTR sequence and co-expressing periplasmic chaperone DsbC that resulted in very high yield of light and heavy chains and improved assembly in the periplasm [39]. These successful studies demonstrated that it is possible to produce complex therapeutic proteins including therapeutic monoclonal antibodies, through proper engineering of *E. coli*.

7. Use of plasmids containing fusion tags to improve solubility

Another strategy to improve the solubility of recombinant proteins is to construct a fusion with a highly soluble protein. Several plasmid vectors are commercially available that carry fusion protein tags. Fusion tags technology can be used to increase protein expression, improve solubility as well as facilitate purification of recombinant proteins. Fusion tags are currently one of the most preferred methods to produce difficult-to-express heterologous proteins in *E. coli*. Some of the most commonly used fusion tags are maltose-binding protein (MBP), glutathione-s-transferase (GST), thioredoxin (TRX), NusA (N-Utilization substance A), ubiquitin (Ub), small ubiquitin-like modifier (SUMO) and split SUMO as shown in **Table 1** [40–43]. Marblestone and colleagues carried out a comparative study to evaluate the expression levels and solubility of three heterologous proteins fused to C-terminus of GST, MBP, NusA, Ub, TRX and SUMO fusion tags. TRX and SUMO fusion partners were found to enhance the expression levels of recombinant proteins as compared to other fusion tags, while SUMO and NusA were found to enhance the solubility of recombinant proteins as compared to other fusion tags [41]. Another study by Braun and colleagues analysed the expression of 32 human proteins of varying molecular weight ranging in size from 17 to 110 kDa using various fusion tags and demonstrated that GST and MBP fusion tags are very efficient in improving the expression levels and also total yield of recombinant proteins after purification was high as compared to other fusion partners [40]. Another study analysed the expression of 40 different heterologous proteins with various fusion tags and observed that MBP fusion tag was very efficient in enhancing the expression levels and solubility of recombinant proteins as compared to other fusion tags [44]. The variations in the data from these comparative studies suggested that the various fusion tags vary in their efficiency for improving the expression and solubility of recombinant proteins, which may depend upon the amino acid compositions, number of disulphide bonds and hydrophobicity of the heterologous proteins. Hence, it is advisable to screen for the most efficient fusion tag for each desired heterologous protein to improve its expression and solubility. One major issue with using fusion tags for improving solubility of heterologous protein is the removal of fusion tags, as it may interfere with the functional activity of the recombinant proteins. To remove fusion tags, cleavage sites are introduced between the fusion tag and recombinant protein, which is recognized and cleaved by site-specific proteases such as factor Xa, thrombin protease or SUMO protease. However, cleavage of the fusion tags can result in lower yield of recombinant proteins. Hence, it is advisable to select the most efficient fusion tag and cleavage strategy to achieve the desirable high yield of authentic and biologically active recombinant proteins.

8. Future perspectives

E. coli is a preferred expression system for production of heterologous proteins due to its well-characterized genetics, ease of genetic manipulation, availability of several plasmid vectors and engineered host strains, low manufacturing cost, high yield of recombinant proteins as compared to other expression systems including yeast, mammalian cell lines, transgenic plants and transgenic animals. However, there are some limitations which need to be surmounted such as codon bias, protein folding and solubility issues and post-translational modifications. Several technological advancements have been made to address these issues. Plasmids such as pRARE plasmids have been designed that contain tRNA genes cognate to the rare codons. Co-transformation of these plasmids would increase the copy number of rare tRNA genes in *E. coli* host and thus would be able to complement the codon usage frequency in heterologous genes. This strategy is very cost-effective and more efficient for enhancing the expression levels of heterologous genes containing large number of rare codons. Solubility and proper folding of recombinant proteins can be achieved by using plasmids that contain genes encoding for molecular chaperones such as GroEL, GroES, DnaK, DnaJ and Trigger factor. Molecular chaperones are known to assist in proper folding of recombinant proteins and prevent formation of inclusion bodies. Similarly, fusion protein tags such as GST, MBP, NusA, Ub, TRX and SUMO can be exploited to improve the expression levels of difficult-to-express recombinant proteins and enhance their solubility. In addition, expression of recombinant proteins in periplasm of *E. coli* along with molecular chaperones provides various advantages such as improved solubility, proper protein folding, easier protein purification and higher yield of authentic and biologically active recombinant proteins. Some of the antibodies that have been approved for therapeutic use in humans such as Lucentis and Cimzia have been successfully produced in the periplasm of *E. coli*, thus confirming the commercial viability of this approach. One of the major drawbacks of *E. coli* expression system is the absence of post-translational modifications such as glycosylation which limits its utility for production of complex glycosylated biopharmaceuticals. Wacker and colleagues discovered a novel N-linked glycosylation pathway in bacteria *Campylobacter jejuni* and demonstrated the successful transfer of glycosylation pathway in *E. coli* to generate a strain with capability to produce recombinant glycosylated proteins [45]. These various technological advancements have demonstrated that *E. coli* can be engineered specifically for each heterologous protein to obtain high yield of biologically active products.

Author details

Ahmed Mahmoud Al-Hejin[1]*, Roop Singh Bora[1,2] and Mohamed Morsi M. Ahmed[1,3]

*Address all correspondence to: aalhejin@kau.edu.sa

1 Department of Biological Sciences, Faculty of Science, King Abdulaziz University, Jeddah, Saudi Arabia

2 Department of Biotechnology, Eternal University, Baru Sahib, HP, India

3 Nucleic Acids Research Department, Genetic Engineering and Biotechnology Research Institute (GEBRI), City for Scientific Research and Technological Applications, Alexandria, Egypt

References

[1] Funnell B, Phillips G. Preface. In: Funnell B, Phillips G, editors. Plasmid Biology. Washington, DC: ASM Press; 2004. xi

[2] Shintani M, Sanchez ZK, Kimbara K. Genomics of microbial plasmids: Classification and identification based on replication and transfer systems and host taxonomy. Frontiers in Microbiology. 2015;**6**:242. DOI: 10.3389/fmicb.2015.00242

[3] Salje J, Gayathri P, Lowe J. The ParMRC system: Molecular mechanisms of plasmid segregation by actin-like filaments. Nature. 2010;**8**:683-692

[4] Rajewska M, Wegrzyn K, Konieczny I. AT-rich region and repeated sequences—The essential elements of replication origins of bacterial replicons. FEMS Microbiology Reviews. 2012;**36**(2):408-434

[5] Frost LS, Koraimann G. Regulation of bacterial conjugation: Balancing opportunity with adversity. Future Microbiology. 2010;**5**:1057-1071. DOI: 10.2217/fmb.10.70

[6] Smillie C, Garcillán-Barcia MP, Francia MV, Rocha EP, de la Cruz F. Mobility of plasmids. Microbiology and Molecular Biology Reviews. 2010;**74**:434-452. DOI: 10.1128/MMBR.00020-10

[7] Aminov RI. Horizontal gene exchange in environmental microbiota. Frontiers in Microbiology. 2011;**2**:158. DOI: 10.3389/fmicb.2011.00158

[8] Frost L, Leplae R, Summers A, Toussaint A. Mobile genetic elements: The agents of open source evolution. Nature Reviews. Microbiology. 2005;**3**:722-732. DOI: 10.1038/nrmicro1235

[9] Sota M, Top E. Horizontal gene transfer mediated by plasmids. In: Lipps G, editor. Plasmids: Current Research and Future Trends. Norfolk, VA: Caister Academic Press, Horizon Scientific Press; 2008. pp. 111-181

[10] Arya R, JSM S, Bora RS, Saini KS. Optimization of culture parameters and novel strategies to improve protein solubility. Methods and Protocols, Methods. 2015;**1258**:45-63. DOI: 10.1007/978-1-4939-2205-5_3

[11] Rodriguez V, Asenjo JA, Andrews BA. Design and implementation of a high yield production system for recombinant expression of peptides. Microbial Cell Factories. 2014;**13**:65

[12] Baeshen MN, Al-Hejin A, Bora RS, Ahmed MMM, Ramadan HAI, Saini KS, et al. Production of biopharmaceuticals in *E. coli*: Current scenario and future perspectives. Journal of Microbiology and Biotechnology. 2015;**25**(7):953-962

[13] Gustafsson C, Govindarajan S, Minshull J. Codon bias and heterologous protein expression. Trends in Biotechnology. 2004;**22**:346-353

[14] Samuelson JC. Recent developments in difficult protein expression: A guide to *E. coli* strains, promoters, and relevant host mutations. In: Heterologous Gene Expression in *E. coli*. Methods in Molecular Biology. 2011;**705**:195-209

[15] Sørensen HP, Laursen BS, Mortensen KK, Sperling-Petersen HU. Bacterial translation initiation—Mechanism and regulation. Recent Research Developments in Biophysics and Biochemistry. 2002;**2**:243-270

[16] Laursen BS, Sorensen HP, Mortensen KK, Sperling-Petersen HU. Initiation of protein synthesis in bacteria. Microbiology and Molecular Biology Reviews. 2005;**69**:101-123

[17] Stenstrom C, Jin H, Major L, Tate W, Isaksson LA. Codon bias at the 3'-side of the initiation codon is correlated with translation initiation efficiency in *Escherichia coli*. Gene. 2001;**263**:273-284

[18] Park YS, Seo SW, Hwang S, Chu HS, Ahn JH, Kim TW, et al. Design of 5'- untranslated region variants for tunable expression in *Escherichia coli*. Biochemical and Biophysical Research Communications. 2007;**356**:136-141

[19] Seo SW, Yang JS, Cho HS, Yang J, Kim SC, Park JM, et al. Predictive combinatorial design of mRNA translation initiation regions for systematic optimization of gene expression levels. Scientific Reports. 2014;**4**:4515

[20] Iost I, Bizebard T, Dreyfus M. Functions of DEAD-box proteins in bacteria: Current knowledge and pending questions. Biochimica et Biophysica Acta. 2013;**1829**:866-877

[21] Linder P, Daugeron MC. Are DEAD-box proteins becoming respectable helicases? Nature Structural Biology. 2000;**7**:97-99

[22] McNulty DE, Claffee BA, Huddleston MJ, Kane JF. Mistranslational errors associated with the rare arginine codon CGG in *Escherichia coli*. Protein Expression and Purification. 2003;**27**:365-374

[23] Yarian C, Marszalek M, Sochacka E, Malkiewicz A, Guenther R, Miskiewicz A, et al. Modified nucleoside dependent Watson-Crick and wobble codon binding by tRNALysUUU species. Biochemistry. 2000;**39**:13390-13395

[24] Tegel H, Tourle S, Ottosson J, Persson A. Increased levels of recombinant human proteins with the *Escherichia coli* strain Rosetta (DE3). Protein Expression and Purification. 2010;**69**:159-167

[25] Carrio MM, Villaverde A. Role of molecular chaperones in inclusion body formation. FEBS Letters. 2003;**537**:215-221

[26] de Marco A. Protocol for preparing proteins with improved solubility by co-expressing with molecular chaperones in *Escherichia coli*. Nature Protocols. 2007;**2**:2632-2639

[27] Ronez F, Arbault P, Guzzo J. Co-expression of the small heat shock protein, Lo18, with β-glucosidase in *Escherichia coli* improves solubilization and reveals various associations with overproduced heterologous protein, GroEL/ES. Biotechnology Letters. 2012;**34**:935-939

[28] Cui SS, Lin XZ, Shen JH. Effects of co-expression of molecular chaperones on heterologous soluble expression of the cold-active lipase Lip-948. Protein Expression and Purification. 2011;**77**:166-172

[29] Levy R, Weiss R, Chen G, Iverson BL, Georgiou G. Production of correctly folded Fab antibody fragment in the cytoplasm of *Escherichia coli* trxB gor mutants via the coexpression of molecular chaperones. Protein Expression and Purification. 2001;**23**:338-347

[30] Folwarczna J, Moravec T, Plchova H, Hoffmeisterova H, Cerovska N. Efficient expression of human papillomavirus 16 E7 oncoprotein fused to C-terminus of tobacco mosaic virus (TMV) coat protein using molecular chaperones in *Escherichia coli*. Protein Expression and Purification. 2012;**85**:152-157

[31] Guzzo J. Biotechnical applications of small heat shock proteins from bacteria. The International Journal of Biochemistry and Cell Biology. 2012;**44**:1698-1705

[32] Ow DSW, Lim DYX, Nissom PM, Camattari A, Wong VVT. Co-expression of Skp and FkpA chaperones improves cell viability and alters the global expression of stress response genes during scFvD1.3 production. Microbial Cell Factories. 2010;**9**:22

[33] Maeng BH, Nam DH, Kim YH. Coexpression of molecular chaperones to enhance functional expression of anti-BNPscFv in the cytoplasm of *Escherichia coli* for the detection of B-type natriuretic peptide. World Journal of Microbiology and Biotechnology. 2011;**27**:1391-1398

[34] Jung ST, Kang TH, Kelton W, Georgiou G. Bypassing glycosylation: Engineering aglycosylated full-length IgG antibodies for human therapy. Current Opinion in Biotechnology. 2011;**22**:858-867

[35] Nelson AL, Reichert JM. Development trends for therapeutic antibody fragments. Nature Biotechnology. 2009;**27**:331-337

[36] Yim S, Jeong K, Chang H, Lee S. High-level secretory production of human granulocytes-colony stimulating factor by fed-batch culture of recombinant *Escherichia coli*. Bioprocess and Biosystems Engineering. 2001;**24**:249-254

[37] Reilly DE, Yansura DG. Production of monoclonal antibodies in *E. coli*. In: Shire SJ, Gombotz W, Bechtold-Peters K, Andya J, editors. Current Trends in Monoclonal Antibodies Development and Manufacturing. New York: Springer; 2010. pp. 295-308

[38] Mavrangelos C, Thiel M, Adamson PJ, Millard DJ, Nobbs S, Zola H, et al. Increased yield and activity of soluble single-chain antibody fragments by combining highlevel expression and the Skp periplasmic chaperonin. Protein Expression and Purification. 2001;**23**:289-295

[39] Lee YJ, Lee DH, Jeong KJ. Enhanced production of human full-length immunoglobulin G1 in the periplasm of *Escherichia coli*. Applied Microbiology and Biotechnology. 2014;**98**:1237-1246

[40] Braun P, Hu Y, Shen B, Halleck A, Koundinya M, Harlow E, et al. Proteome-scale purification of human proteins from bacteria. Proceedings of the National Academy of Sciences. 2002;**99**(5):2654-2659

[41] Marblestone JG, Edavettal SC, Lim Y, Lim P, Zuo X, Butt TR. Comparison of SUMO fusion technology with traditional gene fusion systems: Enhanced expression and solubility with SUMO. Protein Science. 2006;**15**:182-189

[42] Raran-Kurussi S, Waugh DS. The ability to enhance the solubility of its fusion partners is an intrinsic property of maltose-binding protein but their folding is either spontaneous or chaperone-mediated. PLoS One. 2012;**7**:e49589

[43] Young CL, Britton ZT, Robinson AS. Recombinant protein expression and purification: A comprehensive review of affinity tags and microbial applications. Biotechnology Journal. 2012;**7**:620-634

[44] Shih YP, Kung WM, Chen JC, Yeh CH, Wang AH, Wang TF. High-throughput screening of soluble recombinant proteins. Protein Science. 2002;**11**(7):1714-1719

[45] Wacker M, Linton D, Hitchen PG, Nita-Lazar M, Haslam SM, North SJ, et al. N-linked glycosylation in *Campylobacter jejuni* and its functional transfer into *E. coli*. Science. 2002;**298**:1790-1793

Chapter 4

Plasmid-Based DNA Vaccines

Leonardo A. Gómez and Angel A. Oñate

Additional information is available at the end of the chapter

http://dx.doi.org/10.5772/intechopen.76754

Abstract

Plasmids are circular deoxyribonucleic acid (DNA) vectors that can be used as vaccines to prevent various types of diseases. These plasmids are DNA platforms that are usually composed of a viral promoter gene, a gene coding resistance to antibiotics, a bacterial origin of replication gene and a multiple cloning site (MCS) for a transgenic region, where one or several genes of antigenic interest can be inserted. Immunization with these recombinant vectors allows intracellular expression of the encoded antigens by molecular and cellular machinery of transfected cells, stimulating an antigen-specific immune response. This process provides an effective protection against diverse types of pathogens, tumor cells and even allergy and autoimmune diseases. Protective efficacy is achieved by the induction of a strong humoral and cellular immune response dependent on B and T cells. The immunity induced by these DNA vaccines, added to the ease of production, administration, genetic stability, and safety, has transformed plasmid-based immunization into a safe strategy in prevention of various diseases.

Keywords: antigen, recombinant plasmids, vaccines, infectious diseases, immunotherapy

1. Introduction

Vaccination practices have made an enormous contribution to human and animal well-being, becoming one of the greatest cost-benefit achievements in global health. Since its implementation, vaccines have managed to eradicate two important diseases in humans and animals: smallpox and rinderpest, and have successfully prevented a wide variety of infectious diseases: polio, diphtheria, measles, and hepatitis, thus saving the lives of millions of people every year [1, 2].

The vaccination process consists of administering an infectious agent modified to a point where it cannot cause damage or disease but allows the induction of a specific immune response and the development of an immune memory to provide protection against agent inoculated. The same effect may be attained inoculating a part of this agent. Contact between the immune system and the infectious agent's antigens allows the stimulation of this system, activating a specific protective immune response which leads to the prevention of the disease in the vaccinated host. Successful results have been obtained using vaccines based on live or dead attenuated microorganisms (such as smallpox or yellow fever vaccines, or bacterial bacillus Calmette-Guérin strains), or vaccines composed by parts of pathogenic agents: toxoids (such as vaccines against diphtheria or tetanus), protein subunits, or poly-saccharide conjugates (such as vaccines against pneumococcus, *Haemophilus influenzae* type B or meningococcus) [1–3]. Recently, it has been possible to develop DNA vaccines, also called genetic vaccines, through advances in genetics and molecular biology. This method of vaccination is based on the immunization with naked recombinant plasmids, coding one or more antigens derived from infectious agents or tumor cells, which are administered directly into the tissues, generating an antigen-specific antibody response and cell-mediated immunity, conferring protection against the antigens of interest. These recombinant plasmids can be intradermal or intramuscularly introduced or can be also nasally or orally administrated. In these tissues or anatomical regions, plasmids transfect resident cells and use the cellular machinery to express the encoded antigens, stimulating the host's immune response [4].

DNA vaccination offers a series of advantages, including their ability to stimulate the innate and adaptive immune responses. Innate immunity can be activated by recognition of the double-stranded DNA (dsDNA) of the plasmid backbone, while adaptive responses involve antigen processing and presentation in class I or class II major histocompatibility complex molecules (MHC-I or MHC-II) to CD8$^+$ and CD4$^+$ T cells, respectively. Another advantage of DNA vaccines is their safety because the plasmid DNA is stable in biological systems and avoids using whole infectious organisms. Additionally, the ease of manufacturing these vaccines on a large scale makes them more attractive vaccine candidates. These advantages make DNA vaccination an attractive and novel strategy to apply in human and veterinary medicine, capable of providing effective protection against various infectious agents of viral, bacterial, or parasitic origin. DNA immunization is also effective in eliminating tumor cells and protect against allergic and autoimmune diseases through immunotherapy [5, 6]. Furthermore, the optimization of their design, which increases immunogenicity and specificity of antigen delivery, has diversified its applications [7, 8]. Two DNA vaccines against viral diseases have been licensed for horses and fish, one against melanoma in dogs and one growth hormone releasing hormone (GHRH) product for swine [4]. Various clinical trials are being conducted for their application in humans. Promising results made DNA vaccines a biotechnological product that entered the veterinary market already, and it is hoped that soon there will be an effective and safe product for the prevention of human diseases.

2. Plasmid-based DNA vaccine design and construction

DNA vaccines are designed using expression plasmids that are safe for both humans and animals. Expression plasmids are also easily produced on a commercial scale. These vectors are characterized by containing an expression/transcription unit which allows expression of a transgene and a production unit or backbone of the plasmid (**Figure 1**) [4, 9]. Expression units are constituted by promoter/enhancer sequences which are usually of viral origin (cytomegalovirus (CMV), Rous sarcoma virus (RSV) or simian virus (SV) 40 promoters). These sequences regulate antigen expression in various target tissues (high diversity of mammalian cells). This sequence is followed by a MCS or polylinker, corresponding to a short segment containing many restriction sites (sequences that can be cut by restriction enzymes), where the transgene is inserted. Transgenes are found in regions capable of encoding multiple proteins in a single construct, an important advantage presented by DNA vaccines when compared to other platforms. Recombinant plasmids can incorporate several antigens, including sequences with adjuvant activity that increase DNA vaccine efficiency and the amplitude of induced immune responses. Finally, there is the termination sequence called poly-adenylation (poly-A), which is essential for gene expression because it stabilizes the translation of mRNA (alternatively, many vectors contain a bovine growth hormone (BGH) poly-adenylation signal). On the other hand, the production unit or backbone of the plasmid is composed of all bacterial sequences necessary for plasmid amplification and selection. That is, they have

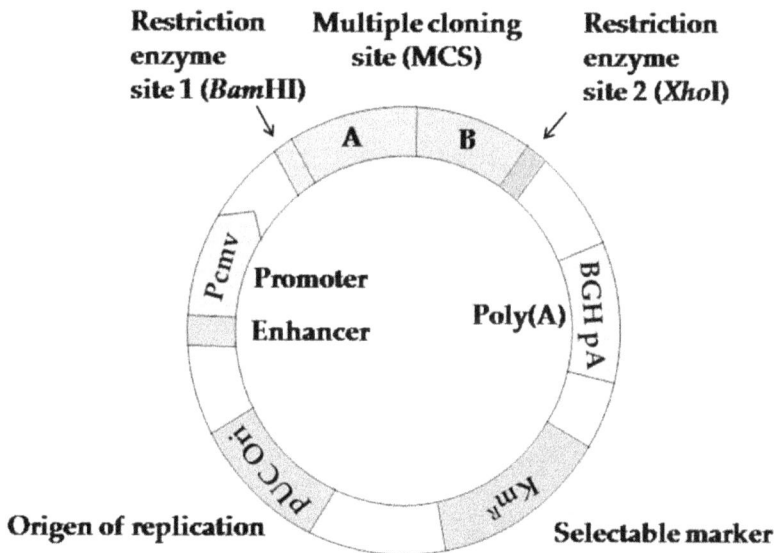

Figure 1. Hypothetical structure of a plasmid-based DNA vaccine encoding of A-B fusion protein. Design of this plasmid is based on Kutzler & Weiner [4] and the commercial pVAX1 vector (Invitrogen, Thermo fisher scientific).

a bacterial replication origin, which usually correspond to a replication origin of *Escherichia coli*, the main bacterial species used for plasmid amplification; antibiotic resistance genes (e.g., resistance to Kanamycin, Km^R) used for the selection of bacteria transformed with recombinant plasmids in culture media with antibiotic (**Figure 1**). In addition, recombinant plasmid replication may also have a replication origin of mammalian, which facilitates replication in animal cells, prolonging the antigen persistence and expression in host cells [9, 10]. Examples of available commercial plasmids approved for clinical use include pVAX1 and pcDNA3.1 vectors (Invitrogen, Thermo Fisher Scientific).

Design of antigenic gene is fundamental to optimize the expression and induction of protective immune response. This design usually incorporates codon optimization to minimize the presence of rare codons and to reduce the formation of secondary structures in the mRNA sequences, preventing translation process inhibition of antigenic proteins. In addition, expression of antigens in transfected eukaryotic cells can be optimized by adding a Kozak consensus sequence responsible for mRNA recognition by eukaryotic ribosomes. Another fundamental variable for cloning antigenic sequences in the plasmid requires that the 5′ and 3′ ends of these sequences possess sites for restriction enzymes (**Figures 1** and **2**). DNA vaccines versatility allows the incorporation of sequences encoding one or several antigens, as well as immune-dominant epitopes for MHC-I and MHC-II molecules, which enhances antigen recognition and adaptive immunity activation. The efficiency of DNA vaccines can also be improved if

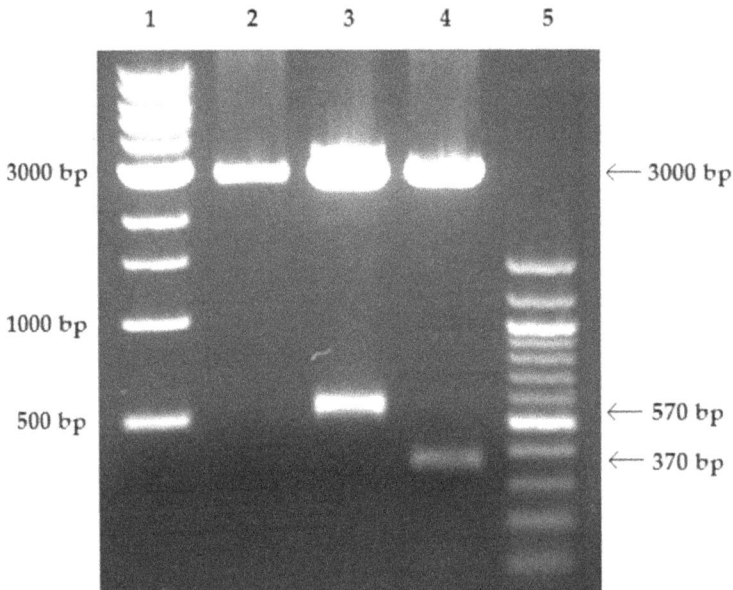

Figure 2. Gel electrophoresis of two DNA vaccines based on the pVAX1 commercial plasmid. These vaccines are digested with *Bam*HI and *Xho*I restriction enzymes. Lane 1: Molecular weight marker (1 kb); lane 2: pVAX1 (3000 bp); lane 3: pVAX1 encoding of a gene (570 bp); lane 4: pVAX1 encoding of B gene (370 bp); lane 5: molecular weight marker (100 bp) [17].

Qualities	Description
Immunogenicity	DNA vaccines have the ability to induce a specific humoral immune response associated to antibody production and a cellular immune response associated to CD4 and CD8 T cells against antigens encoded in the plasmids.
Administration	Intramuscular, electroporation, gene gun, ultrasound, transcutaneous micro-needle, skin abrasion, tattoo perforating needle, jet-injector, or topical patch.
Safety	DNA vaccines are safe since they can revert to virulent forms, due to the absence of pathogens. In addition, several early clinical trials have proved their safety, being well tolerated in humans. Adaptive immune responses against the plasmid do not occur.
Adjuvanticity	Double-stranded DNA is recognized by intracellular sensors such as TLR9, AIM2, STING and TBK1, which activate signaling cascades required for the activation of innate and adaptive immunity.
Stability	They are more resilient to temperature.
Economy	Rapid production and formulation, being highly cost-effective.
Adaptability	DNA vaccines can encode one or more antigens (fusion proteins) from one or more pathogens or tumor cells. In addition, they can code multi-epitopes.
Storage and mobility	Neither requires cold chains, nor special transport conditions.

Table 1. Advantages of plasmid-based DNA vaccines.

co-stimulatory molecules (cytokines, chemokines, or ligands for toll-like receptors (TLR), such as sequences rich in unmethylated cytosine-phosphate-guanine (CpG) [TLR9 ligand] or double-stranded RNA [TLR3 ligand]) are included in the vaccine plasmid [9–16].

After recombinant plasmids are designed and constructed, they are introduced into bacteria using electroporation (electric pulses) or chemical transformation (calcium chloride) methods. Transformed bacteria, usually *E. coli*, are cultured until reaching their logarithmic growth phase, allowing the production of multiple copies of the recombinant plasmid. Subsequently, the plasmids are extracted from these bacteria, avoiding contamination with lipopolysaccharide (LPS), a component of the *E. coli* outer membrane, which is pro-inflammatory and whose administration can produce adverse reactions in individuals vaccinated with this DNA [18]. DNA concentrations obtained are adjusted in physiological saline or phosphate buffered saline (PBS) and stored. Because DNA is a stable molecule, it does not require the use of cold chains, facilitating easier storage and distribution. These are additional advantages of DNA vaccines, which are described in **Table 1**.

3. Cellular mechanisms induced by plasmid immunization

Cellular mechanisms which generate protective immunity against antigenic proteins through immunization with DNA vaccines are being elucidated. Following intradermal, subcutaneous, intravenous, oral, intranasal, or intramuscular plasmid administration, the plasmids transfect resident cells in these tissues or anatomical regions, which are mainly professional antigen presenting cells (APCs, which include dendritic cells, macrophages, and B cells) but also non-APCs. Antigens encoded in the recombinant plasmids are expressed by host cellular machinery, inducing an antigen-specific immune response. It has been demonstrated that plasmids administered orally are transfected by the intestinal epithelial cells (IECs), while in intradermal or subcutaneous administration, plasmids target are skin keratinocytes, fibroblasts and Langerhans cells. Langerhans cells are main APCs of skin, which participate in antigen internalization and migrate to lymph nodes, where they present the antigens to T and B cells. This dermal administration route usually produces a humoral immune response with the production of immunoglobulin A (IgA) and G1 (IgG1). On the other hand, in intramuscular administration, the main immunization routes with DNA are myocytes and APCs, which capture the recombinant plasmids. This route of administration usually induces a cellular response with the activation of cytotoxic CD8$^+$ T and CD4$^+$ T helper type 1 cells [19, 20].

Inside transfected cells, genes encoded in the plasmids are transcribed to mRNA and then translated into proteins. These proteins are processed as peptides by the ubiquitin/proteasomes system and transported by TAP molecules to the endoplasmic reticulum (ER), where they are assembled into MHC class I molecules. MHC-I/peptides complexes are presented on cell surfaces of APCs or non-APCs for recognition by CD8$^+$ T cells. In addition, many of these proteins can be released from transfected cells, being captured, endocytosed and presented by MHC class II molecules expressed by APCs to T CD4$^+$ cells. In parallel, antigen-loaded APCs travel to the lymph nodes where they present MHC/peptides complexes to T naive cells. Soon thereafter, they activate, expand and differentiate CD4$^+$ and CD8$^+$ T cells to various effector phenotypes. In this microenvironment, T cell activation promotes cytokine secretion, along with the release of soluble antigens, activating and differentiating B cells toward plasma cells that produce antigen-specific antibodies. Furthermore, the expression of antigens bound to MHC-I by transfected myocytes activates the cytotoxic functions of CD8$^+$ T cells, causing the release of more antigens [4, 7, 16].

Prior to the activation of the aforementioned adaptive immunity, immunizations with these recombinant plasmids induce the activation of innate immunity. This activation occurs because plasmids are elements of dsDNA of bacterial origin that acts as pathogen-associated molecular pattern molecules (PAMPs), which can be recognized by pattern recognition receptors (PRRs) such as Toll-9 type receptors (TLR9). TLR9 is a receptor which is highly expressed in APCs endosomes. Recognition of plasmids by TLR9 triggers signaling by myeloid differentiation factor 88 (MyD88). This factor, in turn, induces the activation of the interleukin-1 receptor-associated kinase (IRAK) and the tumor necrosis factor receptor-associated factor (TRAF), which activate mitogen-activated protein kinases (MAPKs) and the nuclear factor (NF)-κB (NF-κB). The latter are the elements responsible for the transcription of IFN type I and various pro-inflammatory cytokines which promote cell recruitment, giving way to adaptive immunity activation (activation of T and B cells). In addition, other intracellular sensors for the dsDNA have been reported: stimulator of IFN genes (STING), TANK binding kinase 1 (TBK1) and absent in melanoma 2 (AIM2) proteins. Signaling by STING/TBK1 directs the phosphorylation of interferon regulatory factors (IRF) 3 and 7, activating IFN type I production, while AIM2 receptor activates the inflammasome and the release of biologically active interleukin-1β (IL-1β) [9, 11–13]. These receptors recognize the plasmid backbone, which has an adjuvant effect that induces the production of IFN type I, which is critical for the induction of an innate and adaptive immune response.

Therefore, understanding the intracellular recognition of plasmid DNA and the identification of its receptors has allowed for improving the effectiveness of immune response induced by DNA vaccines. Furthermore, the flexibility of these vaccines allows them to be administered in conjunction with co-stimulatory molecules, cytokines, chemokines, or ligands for intracellular receptors such as TLRs, for instance, the CpG (TLR9) and double-stranded RNA (TLR3) motifs, or the intracellular receptors AIM2, SINTG, or TBK1, whose signaling cascades promote the activation of innate immunity, giving way to adaptive immunity activation. This knowledge, together with the improvements in the targeting of the plasmids to the appropriate APCs, the strategies of 'Prime-Boost' (immunization of DNA followed by protein antigen), and the methods of administration (**Table 1**), will allow to improve the immunogenicity of these vaccines, protecting the host against the challenges represented by diseases caused by pathogens and tumor cells.

4. DNA vaccines used to prevent infectious diseases

Vaccination has helped control the spread of many infectious diseases: polio, diphtheria, measles, hepatitis B, mumps, whooping cough, pneumonia, rotavirus diarrhea, rubella, and tetanus [21]. Protection conferred by vaccination has managed to prevent diseases, disabilities, and the death of millions of people each year. Although the implementation of immunization plans has been very successful in various regions of the world, there are still enormous challenges in the field of vaccinology. Because, in each phylogenetic group (virus, bacteria, or parasites), there are numerous pathogens capable of producing high mortality rates, for example, human immunodeficiency virus (HIV/causal agent of acquired immune deficiency syndrome [AIDS]), *Mycobacterium tuberculosis* (tuberculosis) and the protozoan *Plasmodium* (malaria), alone are capable of causing the death of approximately 4 million people each year in the world [22]. Currently, there are no effective vaccines against many pathogenic microorganisms, and therefore, the diseases produced by them can be disseminated directly or indirectly from one individual to another, producing outbreaks and epidemics with high mortality rates in several regions in the world.

In the search for new strategies to prevent infectious diseases, immunization with plasmid-based DNA vaccines was introduced in the clinical field at the beginning of the nineties. Several DNA vaccines have been developed to fight against viral, bacterial, and parasitic diseases. The DNA vaccination against viruses, obligate intracellular pathogens and highly specialized in sequestering molecular mechanisms of their host cells in order to replicate themselves, has been evaluated. These vaccines were shown to be able to induce an antibody response against several pathogens: herpes simplex, hepatitis B, HIV, and influenza [23–26]. However, to successfully eliminate infection by many of these pathogens, coordination of multiple effector mechanisms of innate immunity and adaptive immunity is required. These defensive mechanisms involve viral neutralization by antibodies produced by plasma cells but also involve the cytolytic activity (perforin/granzyme, Fas ligand, and tumor necrosis factor α [TNF-α]) of

CD8+ T cells for the elimination of infected cells and the production of IFN-γ to inhibit viral replication [27]. These DNA vaccines have also been tested as immune therapy for human papilloma virus, hepatitis C virus, Rabies virus, Filovirus, Flavivirus, and Bunyavirus [28–33]. These preclinical and clinical trials have shown the efficacy of DNA vaccines against various viral pathogens, being safe and well tolerated in humans. Success achieved through immunization with DNA vaccines has allowed the licensing of two vaccines to prevent diseases caused by viruses. These vaccines correspond to West Nile Innovator products developed by the Center for Disease Control and Prevention and the Fort Dodge Laboratories (USA, 2005), to protect horses from the West Nile virus and the Apex-IHN vaccine produced by Novartis (Canada, 2005) to protect salmon from the infectious hematopoietic necrosis virus [4].

With regard to the prevention of bacterial diseases, only a limited number of vaccines are available against a small number of pathogens. In addition, most of these vaccines do not confer complete protection against these pathogens. Vaccine designs depend on the bacterial pathogen lifestyle, which requires that immunization induce a specific type of immune response. Infections by intracellular bacteria are predominantly controlled by a cellular response dependent on macrophages, natural killer (NK) cells, Th1 type CD4+ T cells, and cytotoxic CD8+ T cells. Infection control of extracellular bacteria requires neutralization of these pathogens, activating a humoral response dependent on the complement system, B cells and plasma cells which produce antibodies [27]. Bacterial complexity requires the development of specific humoral and cellular immune response against different structural proteins, toxins, or capsular sugars. The relevance of microbial antigenic epitopes to obtain an effective response is the key to progress in the development of DNA vaccines. Therefore, DNA vaccines are good candidates for the prophylaxis of intracellular and extracellular pathogens due to their ability to induce humoral and cellular immune responses. Their efficacy has been evaluated against intra- and extracellular bacteria such as *Brucella abortus*, *Vibrio anguillarum*, *Edwardsiella tarda*, *Helicobacter pylori,* or *Mycobacterium tuberculosis* [34–39].

The development of DNA vaccines to fight against parasitic diseases is an emerging field. Nevertheless, numerous challenges are involved including identification of suitable antigens due to the complexity of parasite life cycles and their antigenic variability. Some parasites such as *Plasmodium* and *Giardia* have the ability to vary their antigens during certain stages of development, while others such as *Plasmodium*, *Leishmania,* or *Toxoplasma* have developed various mechanisms to escape surveillance of the host's immune system [40]. Nevertheless, to prevent disease by these pathogens, DNA vaccines are a platform that allows integrating various antigens present in different life-cycle stages, or antigens of different subspecies of the parasite, simultaneously. This property of DNA vaccines is essential for the design of effective vaccinations against diseases such as trypanosomiasis (variety of *Trypanosoma cruzi* subspecies), malaria (*Plasmodium spp.*), leishmaniasis (*Leishmania*), or schistosomiasis (*Schistosoma*), which present different life-cycle stages inside the host and kill millions of people every year [41–44].

5. DNA vaccines against tumor cells

Cancer is one of the leading causes of death in the world. Finding effective therapies to combat cancer has been one of the main objectives, since standard treatments such as surgery, radiation, and chemotherapy have had limited success. These therapies are usually effective in early stages but rarely effective in the late stages. Tumor cells may lose the capacity to stimulate or be detected by immune system cells, since they acquire phenotypic modifications. These modifications include the loss of the expression of MHC class I and/or class II molecules, or their ability to process and present antigens due to modifications in the exogenous and endogenous pathways which activate CD4$^+$ and CD8$^+$ T cells, respectively [9]. In addition, tumor cells exhibit a great heterogeneity of mechanisms to evade immune responses, including the recruitment of regulatory cells (regulatory T cells, myeloid-derived suppression cells, and type 2 macrophages), production of suppressors [interleukin-10 (IL-10), and transforming growth factor-β (TGF-β)], and the expression of inhibitory molecules [cytotoxic T lymphocyte-associated antigen 4 (CTLA-4), lymphocyte-activation gene (LAG-3), and programmed cell death-1 (PD-1)], which leads to T cell suppression [45–50]. This immune tolerance induced by tumor cells successfully manages to evade host immune responses, which represents a challenge, but at the same time, their understanding is a path to the development of effective immunotherapy against cancer.

The ability of the immune system to distinguish between normal and malignant cells is essential for the development of effective immunotherapy. The main cells that play a key role in the elimination of tumor cells are innate immunity cells such as NK cells, natural killer T (NKT) cells, macrophages, dendritic cells, and adaptive immunity cells such as helper type 1 CD4$^+$ T cells and CD8$^+$ T cells [27]. Tumor cells express a variety of antigens with potential to produce a tumor-specific immune response. Application of DNA vaccines as a new and novel therapeutic strategy to combat tumor cells has arisen from this property. These vaccines have been developed thanks to the identification of tumor-associated antigens (TAA). These TAAs are expressed in tumor tissues under the control of oncogenes or have been differentiated during cancer development. Many of these antigens are shared among tumors, while others are unique to each tumor [51]. Because some of the TAA are expressed in normal tissues, they hinder the direction of the immune response induced by vaccines, and can generate adverse side effects associated with autoimmune sequelae.

Since the effector responses of T cells against several of these TAAs can be diminished by central tolerance, which reduces the ability to kill tumor cells due to the preexisting tumor suppressor microenvironment, some of these DNA vaccines are designed to express tumor antigens which are fused to co-stimulator and/or cytokine [granulocyte macrophage colony stimulating factor (GM-CSF) or interleukin-2 (IL-2)] proteins, for the recruitment and activation of dendritic cells [14–16, 51]. Therefore, cancer DNA vaccines combine the best tumor antigens with the most effective immunotherapeutic agents. In addition, the antigen choice involves characteristics associated with therapeutic function, immunogenicity, antigen roles in tumors, specificity, expression level and percentage of antigen-positive cells, stem cell expression, number of patients with cancers with positive antigen, number of antigenic epitopes, and cellular localization of antigen expression [52]. These efforts have represented the logical steps for the development of DNA vaccines against cancer, and whose advances have allowed the development of numerous preclinical and clinical trials (phases I and II) against various types of cancer: lymphomas, melanomas, cervical, breast, kidney, and prostate [51, 52]. The success of these cancer DNA vaccines is reflected by the Canine Melanoma Vaccine, product developed by Merial, Memorial Sloan-Kettering Cancer Center and The New York Animal Medical Center (USA, 2007), a licensed DNA vaccine used to protect dogs from melanoma [4].

6. Conclusions

Plasmid-based DNA vaccines are a novel, economic, and effective strategy which induces antigen-specific immunity capable of conferring effective protection against various infectious diseases and tumor cells. Its applications are diverse because plasmids are versatile platforms in which one or several antigens can be incorporated, that allow inducing an innate and adaptive humoral and cellular-type immune response. In addition, their handling, design, and construction are relatively easy to perform. The success of these vaccines has been demonstrated by the number of clinical trials conducted in humans, and by DNA vaccines already licensed in the field of infectious diseases and cancer immunotherapy in the veterinary field. Although there are still many challenges in developing a vaccine for humans, the improvements in design, methods of DNA administration and delivery, associated with new technology, bring us closer to achieving this goal every day. Finally, although immunization with DNA is a successful strategy, its advantages must be evaluated case by case and its applicability depends on the nature of the agent to be immunized, the nature of the antigen and the type of immune response required to achieve effective protection.

Acknowledgements

This work was supported by grant 1180122 from the Fondo Nacional de Desarrollo Científico y Tecnológico (FONDECYT), Santiago, Chile and grant VRID 217.036.046-1.0 Universidad de Concepción.

Conflicts of interest

Authors did not have any conflicts of interest.

Author details

Leonardo A. Gómez and Angel A. Oñate*

*Address all correspondence to: aonate@udec.cl

Department of Microbiology, Laboratory of Molecular Immunology, Faculty of Biological Sciences, University of Concepción, Concepción, Chile

References

[1] Greenwood B. The contribution of vaccination to global health: Past, present and future. Philosophical Transactions of the Royal Society of London, series B, Biological Sciences. 2014;**369**:1-9

[2]   Nabel G. Designing tomorrow's vaccines. The New England Journal of Medicine. 2013; **368**:551-560

[3]   Pulendran B, Ahmed R. Immunological mechanisms of vaccination. Nature Immunology. 2011;**12**:509-517

[4]   Kutzler M, Weiner D. DNA vaccines: Ready for prime time? Nature Reviews Genetics. 2008;**9**:776-788

[5]   Coban C, Koyama S, Takeshita F, Akira S, Ishii K. Molecular and cellular mechanisms of DNA vaccines. Human Vaccines. 2008;**4**:453-456

[6]   Bona A, Bot A. Genetic Immunization. NY: Kluwer Academic/Plenum Publishers; 2000. p. 179

[7]   Iurescia S, Fioretti D, Rinaldi M. Strategies for improving DNA vaccine performance. In: Rinaldi M, Fioretti D, Iurescia S, editors. DNA Vaccines: Methods and Protocols. Methods in Molecular Biology. 3rd ed. Vol. 1143. NY: Humana Press; 2014. pp. 21-31

[8]   Coban C, Kobiyama K, Aoshi T, et al. Novel strategies to improve DNA vaccine immunogenicity. Current Gene Therapy. 2011;**11**:479-484

[9]   Ingolotti M, Kawalekar O, Shedlock D, Muthumani K, Weiner D. DNA vaccines for targeting bacterial infections. Expert Review of Vaccines. 2010;**9**:747-763

[10] Montgomery D, Prather K. Design of plasmid DNA constructs for vaccines. In: Saltzman W, Shen H, Brandsma J, editors. DNA Vaccines: Methods and Protocols. Methods in Molecular Medicine, 2nd ed. NJ: Humana Press; 2006;**127**:11-22

[11] Desmet C, Ishii K. Nucleic acid sensing at the interface between innate and adaptive immunity in vaccination. Nature Reviews Immunology. 2012;**12**:479-491

[12] Kobiyama K, Jounai N, Aoshi T, Tozuka M, Takeshita F, Coban C, Ishii K. Innate immune signaling by, and genetic adjuvants for DNA vaccination. Vaccine. 2013;**1**:278-292

[13] Li L, Saade F, Petrovsky N. The future of human DNA vaccines. Journal of Biotechnology. 2012;**162**:171-182

[14] Melkebeek V, Van den Broeck W, Verdonck F, Goddeeris BM, Cox E. Effect of plasmid DNA encoding the porcine granulocyte-macrophage colony-stimulating factor on antigen-presenting cells in pigs. Veterinary Immunology and Immunopathology. 2008;**125**: 354-360

[15] Barouch D, McKay P, Sumida S, Santra S, Jackson S, Gorgone D, Lifton M, Chakrabarti B, Xu L, Nabel G, Letvin N. Plasmid chemokines and colony-stimulating factors enhance the immunogenicity of DNA priming-viral vector boosting human immunodeficiency virus type 1 vaccines. Journal of Virology. 2003;**77**:8729-8735

[16] Laddy D, Weiner D. From plasmids to protection: A review of DNA vaccines against infectious diseases. International Reviews of Immunology. 2006;**25**:99-123

[17] Gómez L. Evaluación de vacunas de ADN basadas en los marcos de lectura abiertos BAB1_0267 y BAB1_0270 de *Brucella abortus* 2308 en un modelo murino [thesis]. Concepción: University of Concepción; 2016

[18]   Van Amersfoort E, Van Berkel T, Kuiper J. Receptors, mediators, and mechanisms involved in bacterial sepsis and septic shock. Clinical Microbiology Reviews. 2003;**16**:379-414

[19]   Akbari O, Panjwani N, Garcia S, Tascon R, Lowrie D, Stockinger B. DNA vaccination: Transfection and activation of dendritic cells as key events for immunity. Journal of Experimental Medicine. 1999;**189**:169-178

[20]   Shedlock D, Weiner D. DNA vaccination: Antigen presentation and the induction of immunity. Journal of Leukocyte Biology. 2000;**68**:793-806

[21]   Duclos P, Okwo-Bele JM, Gacic-Dobo M, Cherian T. Global immunization: Status, progress, challenges and future. BMC International Health and Human Rights. 2009;**9**:1-11

[22]   Murray C, Ortblad K, Guinovart C, Lim S, Wolock T, et al. Global, regional, and national incidence and mortality for HIV, tuberculosis, and malaria during 1990-2013: A systematic analysis for the global burden of disease study 2013. The Lancet. 2014;**384**:1005-1070

[23]   Strasser J, Arnold R, Pachuk C, Higgins T, Bernstein D. Herpes simplex virus DNA vaccine efficacy: Effect of glycoprotein D plasmid constructs. The Journal of Infectious Diseases. 2000;**182**:1304-1310

[24]   Kwissa M et al. Efficient vaccination by intradermal or intramuscular inoculation of plasmid DNA expressing hepatitis B surface antigen under desmin promoter/enhancer control. Vaccine. 2000;**18**:2337-2344

[25]   Ulmer J, Wahren B, Liu M. DNA vaccines for HIV/AIDS. Current Opinion in HIV and AIDS. 2006;**1**:309-313

[26]   Laddy D, Yan J, Kutzler M, Kobasa D, Kobinger G, Khan A, Greenhouse J, Sardesai N, Draghia-Akli R, Weiner D. Heterosubtypic protection against pathogenic human and avian influenza viruses via in vivo electroporation of synthetic consensus DNA antigens. PLoS One. 2008;**3**:e2517

[27]   Abbas A, Lichtman A, Pillai S. Cellular and Molecular Immunology. 8th ed. PA: Saunders/Elsevier; 2014. p. 544

[28]   Cheng M, Farmer E, Huang C, Lin J, Hung C, Wu T. Therapeutic DNA vaccines for human papillomavirus and associated diseases. Human Gene Therapy. 2018:1-78

[29]   Lee H, Jeong M, Oh J, Cho Y, Shen X, Stone J, Yan J, Rothkopf Z, Khan A, Cho B, Park Y, Weiner D, Son W, Maslow J. Preclinical evaluation of multi antigenic HCV DNA vaccine for the prevention of hepatitis C virus infection. Scientific Reports. 2017;**7**:43531

[30]   Xiang Z, Spitalnik S, Tran M, Wunner W, Cheng J, Ertl H. Vaccination with a plasmid vector carrying the rabies virus glycoprotein gene induces protective immunity against rabies virus. Virology. 1994;**199**:132-140

[31]   Grant-Klein R, Altamura L, Badger C, Bounds C, Van Deusen N, Kwilas S, Vu H, Warfield K, Hooper J, Hannaman D, Dupuy L, Schmaljohn C. Codon-optimized filovirus DNA vaccines delivered by intramuscular electroporation protect cynomolgus macaques from

lethal Ebola and Marburg virus challenges. Human Vaccines and Immunotherapeutics. 2015;**11**:1991-2004

[32] Chang G, Davis B, Hunt A, Holmes D, Kuno G. Flavivirus DNA vaccines: Current status and potential. Annals of the New York Academy of Sciences. 2001;**951**:272-285

[33] Spik K, Shurtleff A, McElroy A, Guttieri M, Hooper J, Schmaljohn C. Immunogenicity of combination DNA vaccines for Rift Valley fever virus, tick-borne encephalitis virus, Hantaan virus, and Crimean Congo hemorrhagic fever virus. Vaccine. 2006;**24**(21):4657-4666

[34] Oñate A, Céspedes S, Cabrera A, Rivers R, González A, Muñoz C, Folch H, Andrews E. A DNA vaccine encoding Cu, Zn superoxide dismutase of *Brucella abortus* induces protective immunity in BALB/c mice. Infection and Immunity. 2003;**71**:4857-4861

[35] Yang H, Chen J, Yang G, Zhang XH, Liu R, Xue X. Protection of Japanese flounder (*Paralichthys olivaceus*) against *Vibrio anguillarum* with a DNA vaccine containing the mutated zinc-metalloprotease gene. Vaccine. 2009;**27**:2150-2155

[36] Jiao X, Zhang M, Hu Y, Sun L. Construction and evaluation of DNA vaccines encoding *Edwardsiella tarda* antigens. Vaccine. 2009;**27**:5195-5202

[37] Hatzifoti C, Roussel Y, Harris A, Wren B, Morrow J, Bajaj-Elliott M. Mucosal immunization with a urease B DNA vaccine induces innate and cellular immune responses against *Helicobacter pylori*. Helicobacter. 2006;**11**:113-122

[38] Bruffaerts N, Huygen K, Romano M. DNA vaccines against tuberculosis. Expert Opinion on Biological Therapy. 2014;**14**:1801-1813

[39] Romano M, Rindi L, Korf H, Bonanni D, Adnet P, Jurion F, Garzelli C, Huygen K. Immunogenicity and protective efficacy of tuberculosis subunit vaccines expressing PPE44 (Rv2770c). Vaccine. 2008;**26**:6053-6063

[40] Carvalho J, Rodgers J, Atouguia J, Prazeres D, Monteiro G. DNA vaccines: A rational design against parasitic diseases. Expert Review of Vaccines. 2010;**9**:175-191

[41] Arce-Fonseca M, Rios-Castro M, Carrillo-Sánchez S, Martinez-Cruz M, Rodríguez-Morales O. Prophylactic and therapeutic DNA vaccines against Chagas disease. Parasites & Vectors. 2015;**8**:1-7

[42] Le T, Coonan K, Hedstrom R, Charoenvit Y, Sedegah M, Epstein J, Kumar S, Wang R, Doolan D, Maguire J, Parker S, Hobart P, Norman J, Hoffman S. Safety, tolerability and humoral immune responses after intramuscular administration of a malaria DNA vaccine to healthy adult volunteers. Vaccine. 2000;**18**:1893-1901

[43] Masih S, Arora S, Vasishta R. Efficacy of Leishmania donovani ribosomal P1 gene as DNA vaccine in experimental visceral leishmaniasis. Experimental Parasitology. 2011;**129**: 55-64

[44] Tebeje B, Harvie M, You H, Loukas A, McManus D. Schistosomiasis vaccines: where do we stand? Parasites & Vectors. 2016;**9**:1-15

[45] Yang B, Jeang J, Yang A, Wu T, Hung C. DNA vaccine for cancer immunotherapy. Human Vaccines and Immunotherapeutics. 2014;**10**:3153-3164

[46] Santarpia M, Karachaliou N. Tumor immune microenvironment characterization and response to anti-PD-1 therapy. Cancer Biology and Medicine. 2015;**12**:74-78

[47] Sukari A, Nagasaka M, Al-Hadidi A, Lum L. Cancer immunology and immunotherapy. Anticancer Research. 2016;**36**:5593-5606

[48] Vinay D, Ryan E, Pawelec G, Talib W, Stagg J, et al. Immune evasion in cancer: Mechanistic basis and therapeutic strategies. Seminars in Cancer Biology. 2015;**35**:185-198

[49] Beatty G, Gladney W. Immune escape mechanisms as a guide for cancer immunotherapy. Clinical Cancer Research. 2015;**21**(4):687-692

[50] Colluru V, Johnson L, Olson B, McNeel D. Preclinical and clinical development of DNA vaccines for prostate cancer. Urologic Oncology. 2016;**34**:193-204

[51] Fioretti D, Iurescia S, Fazio V, Rinaldi M. DNA vaccines: Developing new strategies against cancer. Journal of Biomedicine and Biotechnology. 2010;**174378**:1-16

[52] Rice J, Ottensmeier C, Stevenson F. DNA vaccines: Precision tools for activating effective immunity against cancer. Nature Reviews Cancer. 2008;**8**:108-120

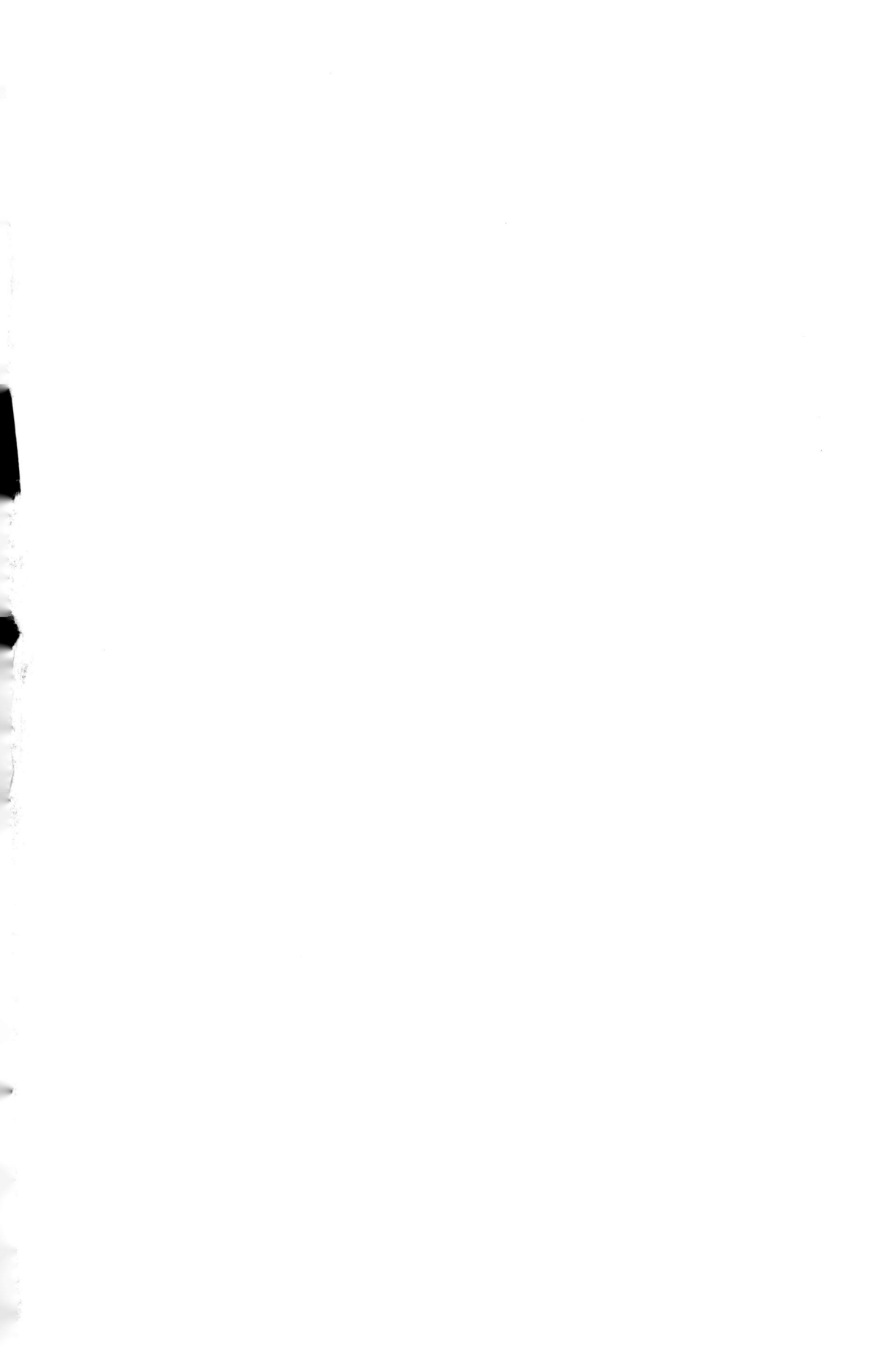

www.ingramcontent.com/pod-product-compliance
Lightning Source LLC
Chambersburg PA
CBHW070156240326
41458CB00127B/5917